DIET WATCHERS GUIDE

by Ann Gold and Sara Welles Briller

Published in Association with *Parade Magazine*

GROSSET & DUNLAP

Publishers New York

LIBRARY OF CONGRESS CATALOG CARD NUMBER: 68-15294

PUBLISHED SIMULTANEOUSLY IN CANADA

PRINTED IN THE UNITED STATES OF AMERICA

ABOUT ANN GOLD

Ann Gold has helped thousands of overweight people to lose ugly fat through the group dieting program of Diet Watchers, Inc., which she founded. She also has taught thousands how to remain slim for the rest of their lives on the Diet Watchers maintenance program which she developed.

She has been a chic brunette with a size nine figure since 1961, but what it means to be fat is her lifetime story. Born a 13-pound baby, she weighed 65 pounds when she was two years old, 155 pounds as a teenager and 185 pounds for most of her adult life. She is only 5′ 4″ tall. Then, in 20 weeks, she took off 65 pounds and she has maintained her new youthful figure, and her weight at 120 pounds, ever since.

She used the diet developed by the late Dr. Norman Jolliffe for the New York City Board of Health to help obese patients lose weight through a nutritious eating plan that eliminates most fats and alters the body chemistry so that it no longer stores fat but turns it into energy.

Ann Gold was a successful saleswoman of mutual funds when she first went on Dr. Jolliffe's diet. But after taking off her own excess fat, she retired and used her new knowledge to slim down her overweight husband and her two daughters. It was while working with her own family that she saw how each person in it reacted differently to the same foods, and she began to experiment with patterns in eating to find the timing and selections that helped each individual to lose weight most rapidly, according to his own chemistry. As they all moved to maintenance she also created her own technique to discover individual patterns for staying slim, and to teach them.

A physician persuaded her to start a Diet Watchers group in Rockland County, New York, where she lived, in 1963. So many desperate people came that she formed another group and another—and still they grew. At first she led all Diet Watchers sessions, but she found herself working seven days a week, so she began to teach other women—all of them formerly obese Diet Watchers—to lead groups using her techniques.

Many heart patients, and people with other health problems that are aggravated by obesity, come to Diet Watchers groups at the direction of their doctors today. "It works," the doctors say simply. Others come on their own because they know that without ugly fat they will be more attractive to themselves and to others.

Ann Gold is not a psychologist (though she did major in psychology at college), not a nutritionist and not a doctor. But she brings to the Diet Watchers program many insights from the three fields and the knowledge that comes from her personal struggle with excess fat.

She also brings the special skill of a good cook. The daughter of a food caterer who supplied fine traditional meals for eight New York restaurants, she was brought up "in the kitchen" believing that good eating is one of life's great pleasures—and she still believes it.

First for her own family and then for the many people of different ethnic backgrounds who came to her groups, she created a vast treasure of Diet Watchers recipes that allow dieters to enjoy a wide range of tasty delights. But she uses only foods and cooking techniques that help Diet Watchers to burn up fat and lose pounds. Without the recipes, a diet for losing cannot be kept over the needed length of time.

People do not "starve" or feel deprived on Diet Watchers recipes. They eat well—of the proper foods, attractively prepared. In this volume she has included her own favorite slimming recipes, and the ones Diet Watchers most enjoy.

ABOUT SARA WELLES BRILLER

Sara Welles Briller has never been a "fatty." Although she has admittedly balanced the scales at a higher point than she liked, she grew up "skinny" and did not begin to fight the usual battle for diet control until she became an adult. For her it began as an occupational hazard. As a magazine editor and writer for 25 years she alternated between expensive business lunches, with tempting high calorie dishes in fine restaurants, and nervous quick hamburgers delivered by the nearest Manhattan eatery straight to her desk where she worked against a pressing deadline.

She became interested in Diet Watchers in 1966 when a friend who had suffered a heart attack was advised by his physician to join a group and lose excess fat. He got a mutual friend to join Diet Watchers to "keep me company." The mutual friend who came along for company lost 50 pounds, persuaded more friends and his own teenage daughter to join, and, because he likes to spread a good word, he convinced writer Sara Welles to come and see what was happening in this kind of diet "group therapy."

After observing the Diet Watchers meetings in White Plains, New York, and trying the diet herself (she took off eight pounds that had previously been stubborn about going), she began to work with Ann Gold to see whether the basic insights and the supports of the group sessions could be translated into book form in order to help all dieters—including women and men only mildly overweight as well as the obese—to lose fat in a healthful, lifelong-lasting program. This book is the result.

Sara Welles was on the staff of *Parade Magazine*, then

on *Mademoiselle, Charm,* and *Living for Young Homemakers.* She was Articles Editor of the *Woman's Home Companion* and a Senior Editor of *House & Garden* and *Printers' Ink,* the marketing magazine. There she developed major articles on communication and also wrote a widely quoted weekly column, "A Woman's View." In addition she has written for *Family Circle, Bride & Home* and *Seventeen,* and is a member of the Society of Magazine Writers. She has covered a wide range of general subjects for women, and written about women for business. She has collaborated on several books, two of which have been cookbooks.

She lives in Larchmont, New York with her husband, Bert Briller, a television executive, and her two teenage children, Joan and Robert.

CONTENTS

About Ann Gold 3

About Sara Welles Briller 5

Introduction: You Have to Hate Yourself *Enough* 11

1. For Men Only 14
2. For Women Only 16
3. For Teenagers Only 18
4. Pills and Other Magic 20
5. "Just Ten Pounds" 23
6. What Happens in Group Therapy 24
7. Setting Your Goal 29
8. Going It Alone 32
9. How to Use the Basic Diet Watchers Diet 50
10. The Basic Diet Watchers Diet 56
11. Ideal Menu Plans 63
12. Frequent Questions About the Diet Watchers Foods 72
13. Maintenance 75
14. Diet Watchers Cookery 77

Index of Recipes 123

DIET WATCHERS GUIDE

INTRODUCTION:

YOU HAVE TO HATE YOURSELF *ENOUGH*

A woman who joined one of our groups once told us, "If I lose 20 pounds, I'll be lovely."

She was thirty-two years old and might be lovely. But she weighed 273 pounds.

We set her real goal together: 135 pounds for her height, and she began a Diet Watchers program to become slim. It took her 15 months, but when she was 138 pounds lighter, she was far more beautiful than she had ever dreamed she could be. She has held her new figure for almost two years and she has learned to see herself as a truly slim person. I think she will remain slim and lovely for the rest of her life.

She had only fooled herself, just like every other overweight person, about her ugly obesity. Fat people always tell themselves they are not as fat as they really are. You may be fooling yourself, too, if you think you are "a little overweight."

Here are the ways you act in order to fool yourself:

1. You look at yourself in the mirror only from the neck *up* (all fat people depend on their faces).

When you put on makeup, if you are a woman, or go to the barbershop if you are a man, your face usually looks fairly good—to you. You may even tell yourself that the little extra roundness makes your chin look stronger. You don't see your face imprisoned in the fat, trying to get out. *You never really see your shapeless body.* You don't want to. If by accident you catch full sight of yourself in a mirror, you look away quickly. You don't watch yourself move and you don't see your *fat waddle*.

2. You wear dark colors. If a woman you buy black and you tell yourself it's because "black is basic." But you really buy dark colors because you think they make you look slimmer.

3. You look for a "special asset" to play up to yourself. You tell yourself you are "pretty," or "smart, hardworking and goodnatured," and so "anyone will take me just the way I am." Or "I'm jolly and a good cook." All fat people depend on this idea of being special.

4. You don't take photographs of yourself.

In the rooms where we hold Diet Watchers group sessions, we cover a wall with pictures of men, women and teenagers that were taken before and at the end of their reducing program. The "before" pictures hardly ever show a fat person *alone*, only in a family group, or behind a table or chair, or with a child. Look at the pictures you have of yourself. How many show you *alone*?

5. You keep putting dieting off. "Today is Wednesday," you tell yourself. "I'll start Monday." Or you go on a diet weekdays, but you break it on Saturday and Sunday. You diet at home but not when you eat out. You may have lost hundreds of pounds but you are not really ready to accept the idea of being slim.

In many cases a husband, a wife or a friend encourages you to really start on the road to slimness. When you do really start, remember this: It took you a lifetime to get fat. You won't get slim overnight.

The Diet Watchers program can help you to lose up to ten pounds the first week safely, and continue to lose two to three pounds a week. You want to lose pounds as fast as you can because the encouragement is important. But you also have to learn to eat in a new pattern that will keep you slim for the rest of your life. The Diet Watchers program is not a fad or crash diet, but teaches you new eating habits you will use the rest of your life.

We have found that most people underestimate their ability. They feel that dieting is too hard. But they sell themselves short. After all, it is *hard* to get a husband, *hard* to find the right wife, *hard* to raise children, *hard* to hold a job and *hard* to run a house. But we all do it. If you want to be slim *hard* enough, you can stick to a diet.

We once tallied a Diet Watchers group for six months. The group collectively lost 25,000 pounds. Most of the members went on to maintenance and are still enjoying their slim figures. But even the "cheats"—people who could not stick to the full program—contributed to that loss.

We urge you strongly to take a picture of yourself. Take it of yourself alone, away from your family. If you can, have it blown up to five by seven inches and then put it up where you will see it often. If you can't do that, carry it as a small snapshot in your bag or wallet. But *look* at it. *Often.* The camera does *not* add pounds. It merely catches you as you really are. You will hate what you see about yourself. That snapshot will convince you eventually to the point where you will hate what you see enough to really start on a fat-losing program.

Happiness is taking your clothes in by four inches.

1

FOR MEN ONLY

Fat men are different "fatties" from fat women. They are more vain, for one thing. Fat men assure themselves that their wives love them as they are. They do know that their wives love beautiful accessories—things like handbags and earrings. But a woman's best accessory is a handsome, slim, well-dressed husband. A husband who wears a watermelon belly cannot be a good accessory to his wife.

They don't make girdles and bras for men, but I have seen men come to our groups wearing girdles. They explain, "I have a slipped disc." I reply, "Oh, misplaced fat?"

One of the successful dieters in my groups was a brilliant attorney who came as a last ditch measure before going into surgery to try to cure severe pain in his back. He had, in fact, already entered the hospital for an operation. He shared a semi-private room with the husband of a Diet Watcher. The husband complained to him, "My wife was 251 pounds and now she weighs 107—and I have to be in the hospital!" Then a beautiful young "girl" came in to visit and he introduced her to the attorney as his wife. She suggested, "You might not have to have the operation if you took off the fat." He laughed, but she proposed that he try it, and he asked his doctor.

The physician was reluctant about the operation anyway. Surgery is so much more perilous for a fat person. It's much longer because of the extra time it takes just to reach through and then sew up all those layers of fat. And there was no guarantee that the attorney would be able to walk, even after surgery. The doctor decided that it could not hurt if the attorney lost weight first and signed him out of the hospital, prescribing a corset to be worn in the meantime.

At this writing, the attorney has lost 45 pounds on the Diet Watchers program, but even more exciting, he has discarded the corset and does not suffer from back pain. For him, 45 pounds made the difference between invalidism and health. Now he is on maintenance and comes in a happy man. His surgeon is delighted too.

A woman will admit wanting to take off weight for her looks. Not a man. "My wife said," or "My doctor said," they explain when they come to us. And when they take off the fat, they act differently too. Most women hide how many pounds they lost—they are still ashamed of how much fat they carried. But a man flaunts the drop. "I lost 15 pounds! See how young I look!" a man will boast.

The difference doesn't matter. What matters is that for your health, as well as for your looks, start on the Diet Watchers program, stay with it until you reach your goal. Remember that your stomach did not grow. You are only eating more of the wrong foods, and you are not aware of it. And as for your wife loving you as you are: You know that a fat man is repulsive to women. In nine out of ten cases, the wife did not marry the husband when he was fat. Did yours?

A little bit of this and a little bit of that makes you big and fat.

2

FOR WOMEN ONLY

Husbands are usually kind, and the endearing things they say to you don't show how they really feel about your fatness. "Fetzella" was what my husband called me. It was an endearing term meaning "my little fat one." "Fatso, I love you just as you are," he would insist. "You're nice and round." But I was round in the wrong places.

"You're just right for me to hold," was another nice try. But he never could hold me. His arms weren't long enough to go around me. On the rare occasions when we danced, it was never cheek to cheek but belly to belly.

I would say, "I have such slim wrists." After I took off 65 pounds I looked at the strap of the wrist watch I always wear—the one my husband gave me after the birth of our first child. I had to cut two inches from it.

I was pleasingly plump, I would assure myself, just as other women say to me now: "I'm not fat. My legs are slim." There were endless other self-delusions: I had big hips. My fat was hereditary. It was my glands. I had big bones.

Today in our groups women tell us: "Having babies stretched my stomach and waist muscles." We say, "You don't stretch your stomach muscles but you do stretch your hands out for food too often." In one DW group we had a woman with 14 children who was ordered by her doctor to take off 75 pounds. Today she looks like a teen-ager, wears a size nine skirt and she can shop in teen departments.

Women tell us: "I have fat thighs." Fat is never distributed evenly. It has only piled up on their thighs. When they take off pounds the ugly fat will come off from wherever it is stored. Many people cannot understand why this happens, but it does.

Fat women are secret eaters, just as alcoholics are secret drinkers. When I was fat I would buy a loaf of fresh-baked onion bread from the bakery and tell them not to slice it—I was afraid they would make the slices too thin. I would run to get it home while it was still warm, cut it in half and scoop out the inside; that part was fattening, I would tell myself. Then I would fill it with butter and gulp it down. And then I would dash to the bathroom to use a mouth rinse so my husband would not know how much onion I'd eaten. The minute he came in, he would ask me, "Did you have onions again?"

I will tell you a funny, intimate thing. My husband never accused me of being fat when I was fat, but he criticized other, small things. Now that I am slim he never criticizes me when I eat onions. When you take off your ugly fat, your husband, who now says he loves you just as you are, will stop complaining about a lot of other things you do that seem to bother him. You'll know then how much he loved your ugly fat.

What you eat in private shows in public.

3

FOR TEENAGERS ONLY

Every phase of life is important, and when you are a teen one of the most important things in life is to be slim. A teenage girl wants, above all, to be attractive to the opposite sex. To the boy who doesn't know she exists. Of course, she can enjoy "hen parties," but after all, they are all girls. If you are a fat teen, you can't have the things you want most out of life at that stage.

I did not have them as a teen, just as I did not have them as a child. I never even had a doll and carriage for the simple reason that I was too fat to be seen pushing a tiny carriage. I looked too much like a *mother*. My mother used to have to buy a ladies' dress in size twenty for me; it just barely fit and she would cut it open to add gussets at the sides, and then hem it to my height.

As a teen I never went dancing, roller skating, bowling or swimming. I was afraid to be seen. I thought that if people saw my fat thighs I would die. Whenever my girl friends went to the beach and dragged me along, I would be the good Samaritan: I would offer to sit on the sand and watch their clothes (wearing mine), and put all their wrist watches on my arms. But despite my shame, I still indulged in food. My poison was cake. "She'd sell her soul for a piece of cake," my mother would say. And I would have. And did.

My first date took me swimming at an indoor hotel pool. They had gray and red tank suits. I asked, *"Do you have a white suit in size fourteen?"* When they said no, I said I would not swim but *watch*. Actually of course, I was a "slim" size twenty, and I knew it—just as I knew they would not have a white suit. But it was my effort to keep my date from knowing my size, and from seeing me in a swimsuit. It was a pathetic date.

A fat teenager tells herself that if she could only get rid of her acne she would get dates. Or if she didn't wear glasses, she would be pretty. Or if only her teeth were straight, the boys would notice her. *But she is looking for excuses.*

I had terrible skin as a teenager. My mother took me to a dermatologist and he put me on a diet. Much as I wanted a good skin, he could not stop me from eating, because nobody cared for me and food was my salvation. It was a vicious circle.

On Saturday nights all my girl friends would go out on dates and I would go to their homes to watch them dress. They would go out and I would go home to cry. The next day they would come and tell me where they went and what they did and it would tear my heart out—and I would eat some more.

Often teens eat because they are angry with their parents. My father used to anger me. He always called me "The Fat One," although I weighed only ten pounds more than my sister. When my mother offered me meat, he would say sarcastically, "Let *her* eat *cake.*" To spite him, I would take cake and hide it in the laundry hamper, and eat it later, blaming him for my being fat.

It is hard to tell the truth to teens because they are at a stage when they *need* to find out things for themselves. But ask yourself: Do the things that happened to me happen to you? A fat teen lies to eat; steals food to eat; becomes a sneak in order to eat. Do you?

You are lying only to yourself. And until you face your own fatness and decide to become slim, you will cheat yourself out of the things you want, as a teen and at every other stage of your life.

4

PILLS AND OTHER MAGIC

The Diet Watchers diet has nothing in common with fads, crash diets or pills. I know because I've tried them all. I was, I think, on every diet ever printed. I probably have lost 1,000 pounds in my lifetime. I am sure that many of you have tried some of the things I did.

Some people like to drink, but I would rather eat than drink, and yet one day I spent $4.98 for a book on a champagne diet, and tried it. I took myself into a liquor store and asked for the cheapest champagne they had and the clerk asked me, "Why, is your mother-in-law coming?" I bought three bottles. It tasted like magnesia to me, but to keep myself from eating I went through two of them, and I assure you it was horrible for me. I could barely make it to bed. I heard my baby crying and said, "I'm coming"—and fell flat across the bed. The next thing I knew, my husband was shaking me awake. I didn't know whether it was night or day. When he got me up, he asked, "Did you feed the baby?" And I asked, "What baby?"

I lost seven pounds on the champagne diet—but of course I could not keep it up and a few days after stopping I gained back ten. Net loss: $4.98 plus the cost of the cheap champagne.

I thought I could go on some special program so I could eat whatever I wanted, so my next stop was taking pills.

I began with a neighborhood doctor—my family doctor had turned me down—who gave me a mild dose of pills just to "lower the appetite." I was supposed to take three a day. I swallowed one with my breakfast juice, the second at one thirty. (I usually did not eat lunch because I was "not hungry enough," so I had coffee and cake instead, thinking it was all right because I'd taken the diet pill.) At four I took the last one. Of course, I wasn't hungry for dinner. But at nine o'clock I ate the entire contents of the refrigerator. I figured that was all right to because I had taken the third pill. It was supposed to do something, wasn't it?

I was seeing this doctor once a week at ten dollars a visit. But I gained weight. I complained to him that the pills were not strong enough. I didn't tell him I was eating cake. He gave me a diet with different colored pills to take just before each meal. I never followed the diet. I actually threw it away because the *pills* were supposed to work—I'd paid for them.

I lost one-half pound. This doctor, I decided, was not for me. I needed one with a better miracle. I found him in a different county. I travelled. He was more expensive—it cost $50 for the first visit at which he did give me all kinds of tests, and $15 a visit thereafter. His pills had all sorts of colors. One was a kind of rainbow pill. I took five of his pills a day and I lost 40 pounds.

But I could not sleep. I was nervous. I felt miserable. I fought with everybody in sight, and when I complained to this doctor about my nervousness, he said, "It's all in your mind."

He added a tranquilizer to relax me. Now I was hopped up during the evenings and I couldn't wake up in the mornings. I felt ill and looked ill, and my husband insisted that I return to our family doctor for a complete physical checkup.

When you lose pounds on pills, you lose muscle as well as fat. And taking diuretic pills or injections dehydrates you; you are drawing needed fluids from your body. You will look emaciated.

In the privacy of our family doctor's office I told the whole story, even about the rainbow pills. He listened, examined me carefully and ordered me to throw all the pills away and see if the symptoms disappeared. I did and they vanished. "What rainbow are you chasing?" he reprimanded me sternly.

"But I am so fat I can't stand myself," I begged. I even asked for surgery to cut out the fat—that is how desperate

I was. He was dead set against pills. He insisted, "Get on a well-balanced diet."

I suffered mental anguish and physical pain. I was a miserable unhappy person who hated myself and everyone else. I can still close my eyes and feel as I did when I was fat. The hate you feel for yourself! Its a feeling of misery. You want to die. You don't enjoy life. You do everything you do because you have to. You feel insecure, inadequate, a failure, a nothing. You think: *I'm not strong enough to beat that little piece of chocolate cake.* I used to go to sleep at night praying to God to help me get up slim. I'd get up as fat as when I went to bed. He couldn't help me.

Many years later, when I embarked on the Diet Watchers program, I lost 65 pounds in 20 weeks. The well-balanced diet kept me nourished and healthy. I loved what I saw in the mirror, and my whole life changed. My marvelous husband became not only marvelous, but also adoring. My children respected me. Everyone looked up to me. I felt like a queen because I ate like a queen, I looked like a queen, and I got the respect of one.

But the greatest reward I ever received came the day I brought my older daughter back to college for her sophomore year. The year before she had asked me to leave her and her baggage in the lobby of her dorm, and she had kissed me goodbye there. Only students, she told me, were permitted upstairs. So I left, eating a candy bar as I drove home alone.

By her sophomore year I had taken off my fat. As we went into the lobby, she said, "Mother, I want you to come up to the dorm." I thought naïvely, "They changed the rules"—until she introduced me to her roommates and then I got the message. "I'd like you to meet my slim teenage mother," she announced. I realized how I had hurt her by being fat. Before, she was ashamed. Now I was slim and she wanted to show me off to the world. . . .

The only magic in weight reduction is in creating a proper diet, as you do on the Diet Watchers program.

5

"JUST TEN POUNDS"

You may feel you don't have the kind of problem I had. You are only ten pounds over, you say. You'd like to be slimmer but is it terribly urgent that you lose ten pounds immediately? The history of all fat people proves that it *is* urgent. You are a potential fat person, because you are not eating correctly. If you don't diet off the ten pounds quickly, and change your eating, it will surely move up to 15, 20, 25, 30, 50–there is no limit to where anyone can go. When you have only ten pounds to lose, you will be delighted with this diet because it will be no hardship.

But I again warn you: So many people come to Diet Watchers and tell us, "I have only ten pounds to lose," and when I put them on the scale, I see they are at least 50 pounds overweight. "What's my goal?" they always ask at that point. If I should tell them 50 pounds, when they have expressed a wish to take off only ten, I would destroy them. I give these people a goal of ten pounds. "Get yourself one size lower," I say. When they achieve it, they become aware that they have "only ten pounds more." But at least they are ten pounds closer to the slim figure they are dreaming about. The truly exciting times come as we move on and make their dream figures come true.

6

WHAT HAPPENS IN GROUP THERAPY

"Group therapy"—weekly group meetings and encouragement by a lecturer—is a cornerstone of the Diet Watchers program. The lecturer always is a formerly fat person who has achieved and kept a slim figure. She is there to give personal attention to each dieter's progress. She herself has won the fight against ugly fat and her success is right there in front of the group to prove that it can be done.

She knows from her own experience how fat people delude themselves, how they cheat, and all the subtle embarrassments and hidden failures that are so discouraging. She can help to find the weaknesses in anyone's application of the program. She helps to solve emotional and practical problems.

But most of all, we find that when men and women who have the same problem get together, to deal with it together, they encourage each other. They laugh together at all the cheating tactics. As they laugh they recognize that the little "secret" excuses and devices they use in order to cheat themselves are common, and human ones. They lose their sense of hidden shame and failure. They feel better able to deal with themselves. And as the despair gives way to confidence, they begin to do much better.

One day in 1965 a nineteen-year-old secretary we'll call Ella joined a group. She was an ambitious girl and highly intelligent—but fat and pimply and terribly shy. A friend, she told me, had been in our program, and recommended it to her. Her first night she sat alone, huddled in the back. At the end of the meeting as she opened her purse to put in her "weighing-in" card I saw that she was carrying a candy-bar. I pointed to it. "Now that you are a diet watcher, let's throw your enemy away." She laughed, and threw it into our wastebasket.

When she arrived at her second meeting, I saw her hesitate at the door before choosing a seat, and finally she dropped down into an empty one next to a thirty-year-old woman. She said a few words to this woman during the evening but not to anyone else, and at the third meeting she sought her out to sit beside. She made a "buddy" out of this woman, but she was too shy to talk with anyone else, and did not see or even talk to her buddy outside the meetings. The buddy was picked up by car at night by her brother who was tall, slim and attractive (and many women in the group were aware of him).

The weeks wore on. The secretary's skin began to clear up and her fat began to melt away and, one June night, the buddy introduced Ella to her brother and the three of them left together.

In September, Ella shyly showed me a diamond watch and said she was dating a "nice man." She did not reveal more, only that he had remarked he was glad she was coming to Diet Watchers and had said, "I could never marry a fat girl." I congratulated her. She still sat next to her buddy, and their relationship seemed warmer but neither of them said anything to me, although her buddy told friends in the group: "Maybe Ella will be my sister-in-law."

By Christmas Ella was wearing a diamond engagement ring—it was official. She invited about 20 group members to a party, including me. I was supposed to watch her and be sure she did not eat. A group member gave her a shower. Two others chipped in and gave her a case of Diet Watchers foods—French-style string beans, mushrooms, tuna, enough to stock a pantry—so that she would never be fat and would always have enough to eat. Ella's shyness with the group vanished. She never told her actual weight but she did reveal that her fiancé had declared he would not marry a fat girl. The whole group began rooting for her. After each weighing-in, she would announce, "Twenty pounds to my wedding!" "Eighteen pounds to my wedding!" "Fourteen pounds to my wedding!" They would applaud.

Then she hit a two-week plateau and she was devastated. "I'll never make it to my wedding!" she cried. The group began encouraging her. "I wish I could give you my weight loss!" one woman said.

A man in the group told her, "I *know* you'll make it. I can see you in that veil, looking so majestic. . . ."

She made it. She was a small girl, only five feet three inches tall. At her wedding in May she weighed 110 pounds and her wedding dress was a size seven. For her honeymoon I put her on "temporary maintenance" and when she came back we worked out a permanent maintenance program so that she could keep her slimness forever. She is beautiful today, and in addition to her husband she has a fabulous job as an executive secretary.

The first thing we advise new group members to do is to find a buddy, and that is also what you, the reader, should try to do. If only one other person agrees to go on the program with you, you've got at least a buddy. You can arrange a place to meet, and work out a plan for following out the program together, and even get a lecturer if by some chance your group of two grows. If not, you can certainly exchange encouragement and check on each other's progress. You can exchange telephone numbers and agree to call each other in "emergencies," as we advise members of Diet Watchers groups to do.

A dieter about to go on a food binge—call her Jane—will telephone her buddy and say something like, "I can't stop myself! I know there's a luscious chocolate cake in the kitchen and I'm going downstairs to cut myself a big hunk of it."

"*No.* You are not!" the buddy will answer. "What vegetables do you have in the house?"

"None. And I've *got* to have a piece of that chocolate cake!"

"You don't," repeats the buddy. "I'll hold the phone and you see what canned vegetables you have on your shelf. Go and tell me right now."

She does hold the wire while Jane goes to her pantry and finds a can of vegetables that she knows are unlimited on the program. She brings it back to the telephone.

"I have a can of asparagus," Jane says.

"Open it," her buddy commands. "I'll hold the wire until you do." And she does just that: She waits while Jane gets the can open and returns to the phone. "Now put it on a plate, or just get a fork and start eating," the buddy orders.

Jane eats her way through some or even all of the can of asparagus while her buddy remains on the wire. By the time she has finished, her self-control has returned. She is fully able to stay away from the chocolate cake.

Happenings like that are common in Diet Watchers groups. Jane will help her buddy in much the same way at another time. They show us over and over again that *if you can get yourself through the single moment of impulse,* which is really what the buddies help each other to do, you will usually be all right—at least long enough to get back in control of your diet watching program. Getting by that moment of impulse is what counts.

Group meetings teach us not to let the size of the total job discourage us. They teach us to take the DW program one impulse at a time, one hour at a time, one meal at a time, one day at a time and one week at a time. That is another cornerstone of the DW program.

One evening at a meeting, a blond girl who had been in the group for five weeks announced that she was giving up. She worked as a hostess in a night club—and she was one of those women who always wears black. In five weeks she had lost 28 pounds and was appearing in bright colors—pinks especially—and was beginning to look beautiful. Her own co-workers knew she was on the diet; they watched her like hawks and they were rooting for her. The cook was even preparing meals for her according to DW recipes, using the restaurant's blender.

But one especially busy night the cook told her he did not have the time to do the extra work of blending. She allowed herself to become embarrassed, tried to skip eating altogether, then hungrily gulped down a hamburger. Looking up as she ate it, she saw her co-workers watching her in shock. It meant the end to her: She had revealed to them that she was not as strong as they thought. . . .

Her group happened to be meeting in a studio used by a dance class and usually, for diet meetings, the chairs were turned away from a long, mirrored wall. But the very next week the lecturer reversed the chairs so that the entire group faced the great mirror. There they sat with their legs spread apart—as fat people always have to do.

The lecturer said to the group, "Look at yourselves sitting

in your chairs. Look at your bodies, not your faces! Go home tonight and lock your bedroom doors and face yourselves in your mirrors . . . and see if you will give up the diet program because you were caught cheating once."

A roar of laughter went up as they saw themselves. Some were not sure whether they were laughing or crying and the blond girl was crying frankly. She did not give up. Sounds hard? Of course it was hard. But today that girl is on maintenance, and looking svelte and absolutely beautiful in her new pastel dresses.

These are the kinds of things that take place in DW group meetings and they prove that even a "disaster" can be turned—with humor and fight—into a new source of strength.

A young woman who weighed 184 pounds told her group one night that while she was looking at her figure, nude, before her bedroom mirror she noticed out of the corner of her eye someone staring at her from the window. She began to scream and her husband rushed in. "A man is on the fire escape!" she yelled. Her husband started for the window, and stopped dead in his tracks. "Did he see you like that?"

"Yes," she sobbed.

"Don't worry," her husband said calmly. "He won't come back."

Today she weighs 116 pounds.

7

SETTING YOUR GOAL

How much should you weigh? The chances are, your answer is far too high and some reasons for your error are understandable. Your mother or grandmother undoubtedly thought that the way to show you love was to stuff you with rich (sweet and fatty) foods. When you were fat, they were contented. If you happened to be a slim child your family probably worried because you were "skinny" or looked "undernourished," although you may have been just right.

And remember all the "average" weight charts we used to see? They were deceiving. Average weight figures are not the same thing as our healthiest weights. The charts prepared by life insurance companies today define our "best" weights because they measure weight by actuarial life and death figures, rather than just averages. As a people, Americans are fatter than they should be. Doctors today are using the insurance company actuarial charts to arrive at best weights. These are the weights we give you here and urge you to take as your goals.

Remember that you have not yet learned to see yourself as a slim person if they seem too low at first. You do not yet know how attractive you can be when you are really slim.

Don't be surprised if your doctor says *he* would be satisfied to see you lose just ten pounds when the chart says you should lose 20. Or if he says, "Twenty pounds less would be great"—but the chart says 40 pounds would be better.

Doctors don't like to be brutal. Besides, they know that

most people hate to diet. An "impossible" demand might be too discouraging. After all, when you come to a doctor with a minor complaint and he tells you to take it easy, don't you let him know that your children or your job won't let you, and he must be living on another planet? So if you don't have a serious health problem, he may decide that it would be an improvement even if you only take off half of your extra fat. He's right about that.

Instead of simply asking him what you "should" weigh, try him this way: Pick a middle figure in the weight range for your frame and height in the charts below, and ask him whether that's a good weight for you, if you can achieve it on the Diet Watchers program.

You will notice that even within each "frame" there is a weight range, and it can go as high as 22 pounds for a tall man. The reason is that it is impossible to put people into simple categories for frames, as though we were all built on an assembly line. You may have broad shoulders and narrow hips—or another kind of mixture. And my idea of a "medium" frame may be different from yours.

Start with your height, be as honest as you can about your "frame," and when you reach your "range," aim for the low end. After you have held it for a few months you will become so used to seeing yourself as a slim person that you'll be better able to decide if you have misjudged your frame. Your doctor can help you to decide at that time, too, and so can the way you feel.

Forget about "age." Teenagers do need to allow for growth but you should always adjust adult eating to stay at your height-frame figure.

Happiness is a size nine dress.

DESIRABLE WEIGHTS FOR WOMEN 25 AND OVER*

(Weight According to Frame—In Indoor Clothing)

HEIGHT† feet inches	SMALL FRAME	MEDIUM FRAME	LARGE FRAME
4 10	92-98	96-107	104-119
4 11	94-101	98-110	106-122
5 0	96-104	101-113	109-125
5 1	99-107	104-116	112-128
5 2	102-110	107-119	115-131
5 3	105-113	110-122	118-134
5 4	108-116	113-126	121-138
5 5	111-119	116-130	125-142
5 6	114-123	120-135	129-146
5 7	118-127	124-139	133-150
5 8	122-131	128-143	137-154
5 9	126-135	132-147	141-158
5 10	130-140	136-151	145-163
5 11	134-144	140-155	149-168
6 0	138-148	144-159	153-173

† with shoes on—2-inch heels

DESIRABLE WEIGHTS FOR MEN 25 AND OVER*

(Weight According to Frame—In Indoor Clothing)

HEIGHT‡ feet inches	SMALL FRAME	MEDIUM FRAME	LARGE FRAME
5 2	112-120	118-129	126-141
5 3	115-123	121-133	129-144
5 4	118-126	124-136	132-148
5 5	121-129	127-139	135-152
5 6	124-133	130-143	138-156
5 7	128-137	134-147	142-161
5 8	132-141	138-152	147-166
5 9	136-145	142-156	151-170
5 10	140-150	146-160	155-174
5 11	144-154	150-165	159-179
6 0	148-158	154-170	164-184
6 1	152-162	158-175	168-189
6 2	156-167	162-180	173-194
6 3	160-171	167-185	178-199
6 4	164-175	172-190	182-204

‡ with shoes on—1-inch heels

* Data prepared by Metropolitan Life Insurance Company

8

GOING IT ALONE

You have no way to create or join a Diet Watchers group, so you are using this book as your "lecturer" and your "buddy."

You must understand, then, that you *learned* your eating problem. Your eating *habits* have made you as fat as you are; they have made you sick just as any poison makes you sick. You did not "inherit" your fat and it does not come from your "poor glands" or your "poor metabolism." Rather, your body has learned to store fat, instead of turning it into energy. And as you lose unsightly fat, your body will learn to tolerate even fattening foods better, turning them into energy for your immediate use instead of storing them.

But first you must change the foods you eat, the times when you eat them, and your portion sizes. These three changes will create new habits of proper eating that will take off your ugly fat and keep you healthfully slim for the rest of your life.

You will use a structured eating pattern that is basic to the Diet Watchers program. Fat people's eating does not have structure; it has usually been destroyed. But without structure you cannot truly see what you eat, and how much. In addition, a clearly timed pattern helps your body to set up a chemistry for losing fat.

Many people do not realize that the foods we eat remain in our bodies for 72 hours before going into the waste track. If you have eaten properly, everything will be utilized as energy. If you don't eat properly, the foods not used up have 72 hours in which to be stored in your body as fat. In others words, your body will not metabolize the fattening food within 72 hours; it remains as fat. Our idea of proper eating is this: When you eat properly, your body metabolizes all the food as energy. When you don't eat properly, your body will not be able to metabolize all of it, and you will gain ugly fat.

YOU ARE A FOODAHOLIC

You are, in important ways, very much like an alcoholic. For example, an alcoholic cannot take even one drink without going on a binge. The same is true for fat people—even for those who have lost many pounds. Once they start on a fattening food, they go on a *food binge.*

A foodaholic *craves* the unhealthy foods just the way an alcoholic craves liquor. He must have the food *right at this moment.* Now—never later.

Foodaholics do themselves almost as much harm as alcoholics and drug addicts, and just like them they hide the truth about the self-damage from themselves. Doctors tell us death rates are higher for fat people than for slim ones. Fat people suffer from more heart attacks, more diabetes, more health breakdowns of all kinds than do slim ones, and it is much harder to help them. Many people in my Diet Watchers groups have been referred by their doctors because their fatness has already begun to threaten serious health breakdowns.

Our diet program agrees with the approches of leading medical authorities who believe that people get fat because they eat too much food (more calories than they expend as energy), and the wrong kinds of food. Medical experts tell us that no one inherits fatness but that fat people *learn* to eat too much. They *learn* the wrong patterns, and they *learn* to have a taste for the wrong foods.

YOUR "APPESTAT"

You have an "appestat" in your body that works like a thermostat to control your appetite. It is your hypothalamus gland, and it regulates your feelings of hunger and satisfaction.

There is no question that you can move your "appestat" up or down. We have found that even after we have retrained it to a proper eating level, if you go back to your old habits of eating in excess, you will send your appestat right up again!

WE DON'T COUNT CALORIES

On the Diet Watchers program we do not worry about calories. We have found that calorie-counting has important disadvantages for most people, and even more for fat people who equate counting calories with "starving" and deprivation. They instinctively resist the idea.

Also, calorie counting is cumbersome. It takes too much trouble and time for most people to pull out a book in a restaurant to add up the calories on all the menu offerings. Even if they do, the count may be inaccurate because of the portion size or the sugars and fats added in the preparation. This same problem exists when you cook at home.

Diet Watchers, instead of giving you calorie count charts and sending you off on your own to figure everything out, uses menu plans and a sound Diet Watchers diet that is high in proteins and low in sugars and fats. The Diet Watchers diet is *not* a restricted one; we give you the sugars and fats your body needs for good nutrition. But it has been balanced in nutrition and timing to develop a body chemistry in which all the foods you eat help your body to burn off your stored fat at your highest possible rate.

When I work with people in a group I am able to adjust our basic diet to help individuals lose more than will be possible in a book such as this, meant to be used by many different people. Still, if you follow the basic Diet Watchers diet here, without cheating, and if you follow the rest of our program in this book, you will lose pounds steadily and learn how to keep them off for the rest of your life.

At Diet Watchers we not only eat the right foods, we also learn to weigh all portions as they are served. The precise portion sizes are vital to diet control because words like "medium" or "small" can mean one thing to me and quite another thing to you. Obviously such a difference between us can throw everything off. After you have learned clearly what the proper diet portion looks like, you will be able to dispense with weighing.

But I assure you now that on the Diet Watchers program *you do not starve,* do not feel deprived, and do not feel hungry. Just the contrary: I constantly have Diet Watchers who have been 50, 60, and 70 pounds overweight complain to me that they cannot eat all the food I want them to eat.

You will find yourself healthier than you have ever been before, while you are losing weight. The reasons are in the nutritional soundness of the diet, which gives you all the foods your body needs and in adequate quantities. All you are cutting out are the unhealthy foods. A Diet Watcher who had taken off 85 pounds told me that for the first time in years he could go about without carrying a secret packet of pills to quell an upset stomach.

NO SAGS OR WRINKLES

You will look as well as you feel. Even if you take off as much as 100 pounds, and no matter what your age, your skin tones will improve and you won't develop wrinkles or sagging muscles. I was in my late thirties when I took off 65 pounds, but I never developed sagging muscles and I did not do any special exercises.

The fear of wrinkles and sagging muscles is common among dieters and is so strong that it can actually get in the way of your will to lose excess fat. I have found that the most effective way to counter this fear is to let dieters see for themselves the strong muscle tone and the youthful looking skin of people who have taken off from 50 to 150 pounds—almost half their previous body girth. Their faces are always an inspiration to everyone in the group when they stand up.

YOU DON'T HAVE TO EXERCISE

We do not use exercise as part of the program, not because we are opposed to it but because exercise will not make up for the poor eating habits that are your problem. In fact, you probably have little energy for activity now because of your extra fat. When you have slimmed down you will have energy to burn for the sports and exercises you enjoy.

NO PILLS OR "MEDICATION"

We do not use pills or medication of any sort on the Diet Watchers program, and not only because there are questions about the efficacy of and dangers in pills. Our goal is different: We aim to reeducate you and your "appestat"

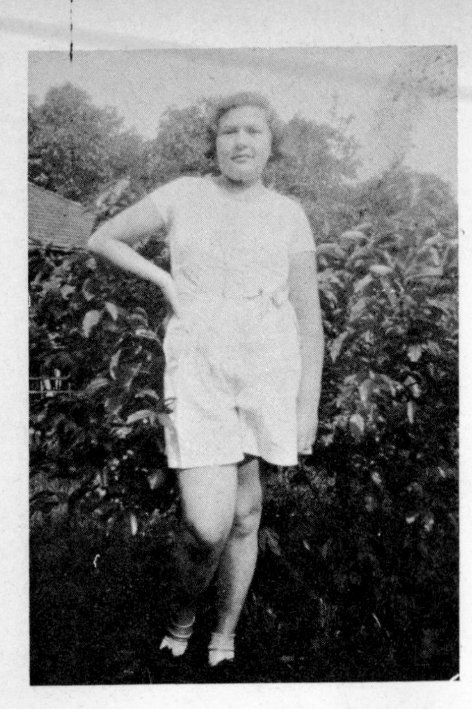

Ann Gold as a teenager.

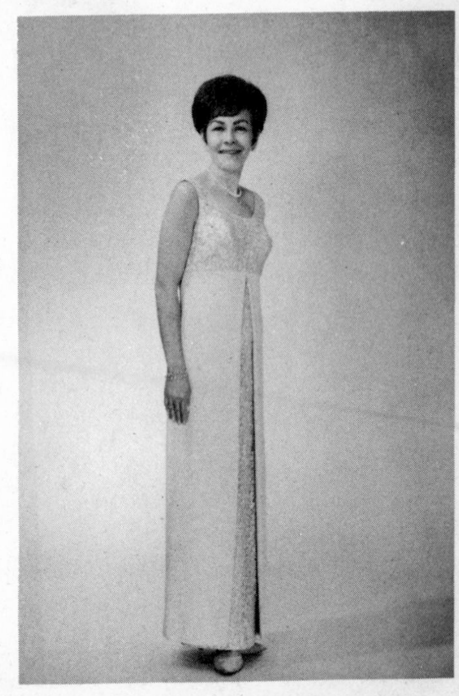

Ann Gold today.

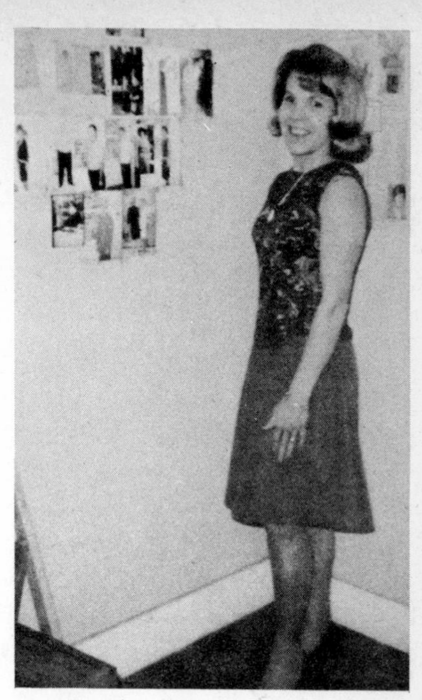

Joan Albonese, a Diet Watcher lecturer who lost 60 pounds under the program, inspects some "before-and-after" snapshots on the wall of a Diet Watchers studio. Among them is one of Joan herself (below) before she became a Diet Watcher.

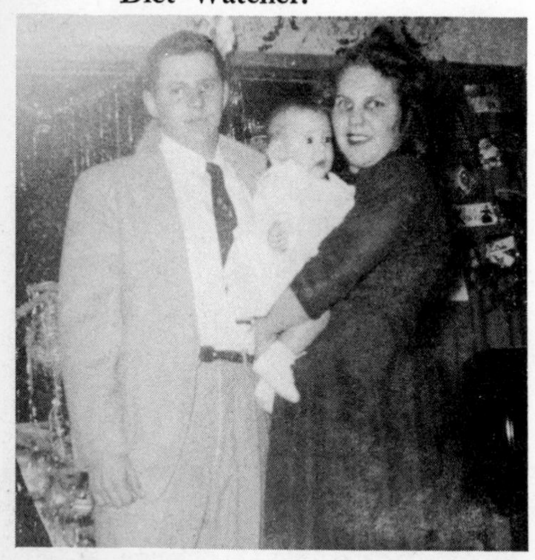

to a healthy eating pattern that will keep you slim for the rest of your life. No pill can do that. You achieve it only by learning new eating habits.

SEE A DOCTOR

It is only sensible to have a doctor's checkup before putting yourself on *any* diet. If there is any reason why you should not go on a diet, only your doctor can tell you. We do not accept people with a health problem in any Diet Watchers group without a doctor's written approval, and you should give yourself the same protection.

DON'T "CRASH" DIET

Diet Watchers opposes "crash" dieting, not so much because of the dangers to health and the starvation regime that no one can hold for long, but because our goal is to develop new eating patterns *while you are losing your ugly fat.*

Remember, once you attain your best weight you will need to find a maintenance pattern you can stay with forever, one that allows you to enjoy good eating and to have your slim figure too. A crash diet may take off pounds quickly but you cannot live with it. And as soon as you return to your old eating patterns you will certainly put that ugly fat right back on.

At the same time, Diet Watchers believes in taking off your excess fat just as fast as you healthfully can, primarily to combat your own discouragement. Time *is* important. For example, if you have 50 pounds to lose, an average drop of half a pound a week means that you have to fight discouragement for 100 weeks. But a two-pound average weekly loss on the Diet Watchers' program is healthy, and cuts your dieting time to only 25 weeks.

Of course, the more overweight you are, the more you can lose healthfully. As you approach your goal, you will show smaller losses on the same diet, and that is normal.

HOW TO GAUGE YOUR WEEKLY LOSSES

When you don't cheat on the basic Diet Watchers diet *you can expect to lose up to seven pounds the first week* (depending on how fat you are now) and an average of two pounds a week thereafter until you come very close to your goal, when it may drop to one pound a week. Working with an individual in a group, I usually adapt the basic diet to his chemistry as I observe him, and I can help people lose fat at a higher average rate. I adapt both the foods and the time of day when they are eaten. However, this of course is impossible in a book meant to be read by many. You will do best to follow the basic diet. It will take you a little longer than it takes us, but you will surely reach your goal.

PLATEAUS: WHAT THEY ARE AND HOW TO HANDLE THEM

Everyone who diets experiences the plateau—a period when you stop losing weight, even though you are following the same diet that has been paring off pounds. You simply stay at that level, and it can go on for two or three weeks. A plateau is suprising, bewildering, frustrating. But what is happening is normal, and it is important that you understand it.

Your body has been working hard to burn off its stored fat as energy. It works harder doing this than it does turning food into energy. You stop losing weight because your body must rest.

While your body is at rest, however, something else—also quite wonderful—takes place. Your body rēdistributes your fat and you will find that although you are not losing weight, your measurements are changing. You are losing inches. Your figure improves. These are the times when fat "miraculously" comes off the thighs and hips of women who thought that they were just unfortunately "shaped" that way.

These are the times also, however, when many people become discouraged and give up their diets. The most important thing about a plateau is not to give up. You must continue with the Diet Watchers diet right through it.

I think probably the toughest plateau I ever saw happened to a girl in one group who had dropped 35 pounds and suddenly stopped losing. She did not lose another pound for three weeks. When she got on our scale and saw that her weight was still the same, she would burst into tears. I used every technique I know to reassure her. "Fine! You are leveling off. Don't give up now," I would urge.

"But I'm losing inches!" she would say. "Why doesn't it show on the scale?" After three weeks of this, she did begin to show pound losses again.

I have found that some people hit plateaus at every 25–35 pound loss, while others can go for 50 pounds before they level off. But wherever your plateau, if you stay on the diet, once your body has rested sufficiently it will start functioning on the fat-burning cycle again. Just don't give up the diet.

YOUR "FRIENDLY" ENEMIES

Since you are going on the Diet Watchers program while living with your fat friends, it is you and this book against them. Let's start with the toughest of them all—your fat grandmother, or your mother who comes with her shopping bag to buy love at your house. She comes bearing cookies and goodies that she thinks are giving you love but that, to you, are *poison*. You have to do something about grandmother or mother, and the first thing is to run a *different kitchen* in your home from the one she ran in hers. Why continue to eat what is poison to you? Why pass a taste for these illness-producing habits to *your* children?

If you are eating at grandma's house and she must serve in her usual way, or pushes foods that are damaging to you, *learn to pass up*. Choose from what is offered. Choose the lean instead of the fat, the right instead of the wrong, the foods that are your friends and not your enemies. If you hate to pass up a "treat," remind yourself at this instant just how you will hate what you see on your scale the next time you weigh yourself.

Often at meetings we hear the common argument: "I can't offend my mother, or grandma." You are merely kidding yourself. Insist on eating what you want, not what others want you to eat. If you are not ready to diet, you worry about other people's "feelings." But when you are truly ready to be slim, you worry about yourself. The same holds true for your friends who "entertain" you by pushing poison into you.

Do you get embarrassed when you refuse? People who are ill do not feel ashamed because they cannot have foods that do them harm. You are suffering from an illness. You are "allergic" to food. The "treat" being served will cause you to break out in fat all over your body.

Are your friends *friends?* Let us see. How many of them are overweight and what is *their* stake in keeping you fat? Remember that in group therapy, you get big support by surrounding yourself with new friends who, like you, have a commitment to becoming *slim.* You all have a stake in the success of your common goal. You may as well face the fact that your new slimness may truly threaten your fat friends.

In one of our groups, a twenty-four-year-old girl who was a secretary weighed 165 pounds when she started with us, and she wore a size eighteen dress. She had as a good friend in her office another secretary who claimed to wear size twelve. Our dieter envied the other girl. This friend teased her mercilessly about the new diet when they out together for lunch and on every other possible occasion.

But one day our Diet Watcher had her revenge. Wearing a new dress, she asked her friend if she would look down into the back of it. "I feel scratchy," she said.

"It must be that *diet* you're on," her friend replied solicitously, as she unhooked the back and pulled down the zipper to find the trouble. Sure enough, she found something. The size tag was still there. The friend pulled it out. *"It's a size twelve!"* she fairly shouted.

"Yes. And it's loose," our dieter said coolly.

This "friend" has hardly spoken to her since, but that is not the entire story. The Diet Watcher is now wearing a size nine—the proper size for her height and frame—and she is much slimmer than her office mate who, she now realizes, could not possibly wear size twelve dresses but had to be size fourteen or sixteen. When she herself was squeaking into a size eighteen dress, she could not tell the difference.

If you look for support from fat friends when you take off ugly pounds you will be disappointed. You are smarter to watch out for their *discouragements.*

"Stop *now* or you'll look terrible!" (a "friend").

"Now you're drawn and haggard!" (your mother).

"Eat—they're starving in India!" (your grandmother).

"Eat—it costs money" (mama?).

One pretty young woman reported to a DW group that her mother now called her "Pruneface." To reassure her that, on the contrary, she looked lovely, the lecturer asked her to stand before the group. "We are all fat, but we are honest," the lecturer urged. "Let us see if they think your face is like a prune."

The people in the group cried out, "Don't listen to her!"

"Friends"? At Diet Watchers we call them *friendly enemies.* They feel that they are losing you when you become slim and look better than they do. In fact, for any number of reasons that we won't bother to examine here, they will not only try to ridicule or to frighten you, they may actually try to force you to eat the foods that keep you fat by showing displeasure when you refuse. If you lose some of these fat "friends," you will gain new slim ones, people who are much better for you, as you move into a new slim world.

SELF-PITY AND OTHER SELF-DELUSIONS

Many fat people eat and drink their poisons when they are with friends because they feel sorry for themselves. Watch yourself closely the next time you break your own resolve. Don't you feel that twinge of self-pity? If you are grieving for yourself because you cannot eat more, remember that you are suffering from "fat eyeballs." This disease of obesity makes all portions look small. When you have lost your fat and are on maintenance, you'll find that your eyeballs will be slimmer, too, and the ordinary portions will look correspondingly larger.

Or do you feel self-pity because you can't have what the rest of the crowd is enjoying? You may give in to a common switch-delusion. Watch it in action the next time you are eating in a group with other fat people. Watch how one of them announces daintily, after most of the crowd has ordered strawberry shortcake: "Well, *I'll* have a *plain* piece of Danish."

She feels sorry for herself but proves to herself and to the others that she has self-discipline. But her plain Danish pastry has practically the same number of calories as the luscious strawberry shortcake her friends are enjoying. So who is being fooled, and who is doing the fooling?

THE "RESTAURANT PROBLEM"

That brings us to the "restaurant problem." Most restaurants today offer fish and lean meats for lunches and dinners.

Most times you can order and get food exactly as you want it. Without mayonnaise, on lettuce with the proper vegetables, with one slice of white bread, toasted or not—but without butter, if you ask for it that way. You can get buttermilk, tea or coffee. You can bring your own saccharin.

What stops you?

You don't want to reveal that you are dieting—you who may be drowning in pounds of fat that shows all over you like a fatty *tumor* spread all over your body? Do you hide this from others because you hide it from yourself?

Are you embarrassed because you are demanding a little extra time or attention from the waiter or waitress?

Or afraid of the attention from others if the waiter should get unpleasant? People who are serious about dieting remember that *they* are paying for what they eat in public places, and if they accept second-rate service, they only deserve second-rate service. The food they want is there and can be served to them as they want it.

HOW TO HANDLE A DIFFICULT WAITER

If the waiter or waitress gets obstreperous, you can handle it easily. At one of our early working sessions we went at lunchtime to a well-known variety store to order from the take-out counter. A young waitress approached and we asked for a tuna salad on lettuce, one slice of white bread, unbuttered, and one black coffee. Our waitress pointed to the wall menu card. "No tuna salads. Just sandwiches."

"Can't you make up a salad?" we asked.

"Sandwiches," the girl repeated blankly.

"Don't you have a paper plate?"

The girl's eyes widened but she admitted that she had paper plates.

"Don't you have lettuce?"

". . . Well, yes." The girl was irritated now.

"Don't you have tuna?"

With a little cry of exasperation, the waitress fled to the other end of the counter and told her supervisor—a slightly older girl—the horrible thing being demanded. We could see the supervisor nod her head in a way that meant to let us have it. The waitress controlled herself, took a seven-inch paper pie plate, put on some lettuce leaves, a serving of tuna, covered it carefully under wax paper, added a slice of plain toast and poured us a cup of black coffee. Our order was no harder to prepare than a sandwich, although she bit her lips in silent fury as she handed it across the counter and took our money. Thereafter we asked for the same order every time we came in, and she gave it to us without a question.

But that first time, as we ate, we analyzed what had taken place.

Most people would have taken the sandwich just because they would be embarrassed about the attention the argument would get. But we took the offensive. We showed her how to do it, and that made *her* feel inadequate. *She* was embarrassed, and that was why she was angry. But why shouldn't *we* have authority over what *we* pay for?

You can avoid conflict in restaurants—especially with a waiter in a fancy place when you are having dinner out—by announcing that you must have your order *exactly* as you want it, without certain foods, because you have an allergy and could become very ill immediately. You will be amazed at how beautifully it works. A restaurant dreads the idea that anyone might become ill while eating there. You will get exactly what you order, served with extreme care and attention—*and no argument.*

YOUR "LITTLE CARE" PACKAGE

If you know you will truly be in a place where you cannot obtain the proper food, you can carry a Diet Watchers "Little Care" package with you. This makes a full and satisfying lunch and is small enough to fit into an ordinary handbag, and there is no reason why you cannot eat it, in an emergency, at your desk, in the park, or in the ladies' lounge.

A television producer in one Diet Watchers group sent me a card from a business trip on the red carpet flight from New York to Los Angeles, to tell me that the multi-million dollar plane he was on did not carry a can opener, and so he used his pocket knife to open a can of tuna for a Diet Watchers meal, while his co-passengers watched him in awed fascination. He enoyed their awe, he reported.

Many a woman Diet Watcher has taken off ugly fat by eating a DW Little Care package each day in the ladies' room, instead of swallowing unhealthy food she should not have.

To make a Little Care package, put 3¾ ounces of tuna on half a slice of toasted white bread, and cover with the second half-slice. It makes a thick half-sandwich and you'll have a few nibbles of tuna to eat separately. Or put the tuna into a small paper bowl, cover with foil, and have the slice of bread on the side. Add lettuce and any unlimited vegetable you like—cucumber, red or green pepper, pimiento, cauliflower—in any amount that will satisfy you. Put everything in a small plastic bag. Buy coffee or tea to go with it, if you want—and put the money you save toward your exciting new wardrobe of smaller-sized clothes.

Prepare your Little Care package at night, so that it is ready in the morning when you are in a rush. My habit is so well established that it is easy for me to get it ready each evening after dinner, before I clean up the kitchen.

I first devised the Little Care package to help me solve the problem of my own lack of control. I used to eat anything that wasn't nailed down. I never got past the cake counter at the door when I walked into a restaurant. I knew I needed protection from temptations I couldn't handle when I was dieting, because I wasn't strong enough then to fight my enemy. I decided that the only way I could win was not to see fattening food when I was hungry. I carried the Little Care package with me for lunch, and after I started using it I found it was also wonderfully useful, because I was selling mutual stock at the time and did not know where I might be at lunchtime any day. With my package it did not matter. I could have my proper lunch at the same time each day, no matter where I was.

You may be different. You may have the self-control to find the food you should in a restaurant (I can, now) and get it. After the first time, the people who work in restaurants will help you. But if you are like me, or if you are frequently forced to eat in a place where you cannot find the proper food, use Little Care.

Sometimes people tell me they can't go to work carrying a package. That is not true. If you can't fit it into your present handbag, get one that will hold it. I used to drive to work in a carpool with five men when I was fat. Whenever I arrived they would shout, "Here she comes . . . *shift!*" I carried my Little Care package and also emergency cans of unlimited vegetables and a can opener all in a shopping bag. They would ask, "What have you got there?" I'd say, "Food." "You don't eat *enough?*" they would ask. But I knew what I was doing. I knew that if I could do other hard things in life, I could do this.

As time went on and I began to lose fat, they had more room on the carseat, and they would ask, "Hey, you losing weight?"

One night when coming home, I opened a can of asparagus in the car. They broke up. I drank the juice and they laughed. "Will you eat the can, too?" I put the empty can in my shopping bag calmly and I felt good, because now they were also saying, "Hey, we have room now for another passenger!" I replied, "Fine! We'll save money!"

I even carried a plastic bag of powdered skim milk and some liquid sweetener with me. I would go into a restaurant and give the counterman the bag of powdered skim milk and ask him to put it through his blender to make a Diet Watchers malted. He could charge me his regular price, I'd say. He would ask, "Do you call this a *malted?*" But he'd make it, and not charge me, although I would have been happy to pay.

There were times too when I gave a counterman a small can of tuna (in those days you could not find tuna or salmon salads made without mayonnaise), ask him to put it on a bed of lettuce and offer to pay his regular price. "I have an allergy," I would explain. "I break out all over." I did not add "with fat." He would always make it my way, and kindly not charge me.

THE DANGER IN EATING ALONE

When you are alone and eating at home, you may be tempted by the demon of just plain laziness, the feeling that you don't want to "bother" cooking for yourself. It is common. Many people will cook for hours to please or to impress others, but they avoid preparing a meal for themselves.

Yet *you* are the most important person in your world. And you are the center of the world for your children, and your husband or wife. Value yourself enough to take the trouble to prepare a meal for yourself. Use a proper place mat and make the table look pretty. Take the trouble to set a meal for an important person—*you*—because then you will be far less likely to give way to self-pity and to break your diet.

WHEN YOUR SELF CONTROL IS SLIPPING

Take action.

1. Call your diet buddy.
2. If you can't, call anyone and talk of anything but food.
3. If that is not possible, find your can opener, pull out a can of any unlimited vegetable and *start eating*. Once you have a can of vegetables in you, your mind *and your control* will begin to function again.

Remember that a food binge is just like an alcohol binge. If you can stave off the moment of temptation, you will be all right.

PLAN AHEAD FOR YOUR PRIVATE WITCHING HOURS

Everybody has a witching hour—a special time of day when his self-control is at its lowest and he is most likely to cheat. For some people it comes at 3:30 and for many it is when they sit down to enjoy TV—and bring out the treats. Prepare for it. Arm yourself ahead with foods you like that are good for you. My witching hour comes after dinner and so when I was losing 65 ugly pounds I would prepare a big pot of French-style string beans, bean sprouts, mushrooms and Chinese cabbage, and let it keep warm on the stove. When I wanted to eat I would put some in a bowl, mix in a bit of English mustard—and enjoy a Chinese dinner of unlimited vegetables.

Then I'd have my fruit, and my last four ounces of daily skim milk in a malted, DW style. I was contented because I was busy eating almost all night long, and this was marvelous food to put in my body.

WHEN YOU HAVE CHEATED

The most important thing to remember about cheating is that just because you fell down, it doesn't mean you have to lie there. You will find it rough, but pick yourself up, brush yourself off and get back on your program. And do it *immediately*. Never say, "I cheated for lunch, so I'll cheat for dinner." Get back now.

Don't worry about what slim people think. Remember that

fat people all have the same mental and physical pain and only a fat person knows what another fat person endures. *Get back on the program at the very next meal.*

NEVER SKIP A MEAL

At Diet Watchers meetings we hear men and women 150 pounds overweight insist that they eat only one meal a day. They are telling the truth, but that single meal, in little nibbles, goes on all day.

Other fat people starve all morning and afternoon but from dinnertime on they never close their jaws. Both of these types cannot control their obesity because they do not have a clear eating pattern. True self-control comes when you eat in a clear design.

Sometimes emotional blocks hang you up. I used to feel that breakfast made me nauseous—until I discovered, in 1961, that the *fear* that eating made me fat caused the nausea. *When I had absolute conviction that a proper breakfast would help me to lose fat, the nausea disappeared.* Today my breakfast invariably consists of half a grapefruit, a poached egg on toast, and coffee.

You don't get ahead of the game by skipping a meal. On the contrary, you get yourself so famished that you wolf down the wrong food, and too much of it. You put yourself in a position where self-control is much harder, and you fail also to lay the foundation for a lifetime maintenance diet.

There is one other important reason why you should never skip a meal or let more than five hours go by without eating on the Diet Watchers plan: *Skipping can actually cause you to gain weight.* This is easy to understand if you remember that the proper foods burn fat to turn it into energy. A neutritionally well-balanced diet, on the proper time schedule, gears your body to turn fat into energy. It does not store fat. If you fail to take in the foods that burn the fat, your body will not be able to do this job and will have to store the fat instead. The proper food is vital because it helps to burn the fat and gives you tremendous amounts of energy.

So don't skip meals and don't delay them. Eat in a well-defined pattern that you can control.

ENJOY DIETING

You don't help your diet by depriving yourself of eating pleasure while you lose ugly fat, so don't try to cut out the non-sugar sweet treats and desserts that are part of the program. Develop a sense of adventure in trying the Diet Watchers foods. Keep a sense of humor about the things that happen to you while dieting. In group meetings, humor helps; laughter is one of the things we use to bring people together. Laughter helps fat people to identify with the lecturer. We have good times at our Diet Watchers meetings.

I always tell people about myself. I tell of my own secret eating devices, my old ways of cheating. I used to hide in the bathroom to eat the chocolate cake I had hidden in the hamper. I still remember, for example, how once when my mother threw dirty napkins on top of my cake I dug it out and not only gobbled it up but then I licked at the napkins to get every last bit of chocolate. I tell people this without shame because it helps them to see that if I, who did the same ridiculous things they do, could take off 65 pounds and keep them off—and enjoy life as I do—so can they.

It's not how old you are that counts but how young you look.

9

HOW TO USE THE BASIC DIET WATCHERS DIET

By now I expect that you have already flipped pages to see what the basic diet is like. To make it work you need to employ a few new techniques—none of them hard. I introduce them as fast as new members can put them into use. You should plan to start using them at once, together with the diet.

If you try to introduce Diet Watchers cookery to your whole family at once, you may have rebellion on your hands—and this can discourage you. Nobody likes to change. If others are slim, they don't need this diet. Even if they are fat, it was you who joined a group or bought this book, not they. It is sensible to try new dishes on them, but not to force them to eat any they don't like. Cook for yourself separately, and keep leftovers for other meals so that nothing gets wasted.

Here are the few new techniques you need to make the basic diet work.

WEIGH ALL PORTIONS

Until you learn how to judge the size of portions, use a scale to weigh all meat, fish and the sugared vegetables in order to guarantee that you eat just the proper amount each time. Buy a postage-stamp scale (cost: about $3) that shows ounces; use an aluminum foil pie plate to hold the food.

You are in for a pleasant surprise if you expect you'll have to cut your portions. You will eat larger amounts of vegetables than you expected, and more meat, too—you will be amazed at how much more meat. Many people eat smaller portions than they should because they are geared to a "cut-your-portions!" idea. Then they fill up on the fattening dessert course.

This weighing also trains your eye so that after a while you will accurately estimate size when someone else fills your plate, and can judge how much you should eat and how much to leave. While you are learning portion sizes, get out your measuring cups to see just how high skim or buttermilk drinks come in your regular glasses, and how high four ounces of juice come in your own juice glasses.

KEEP RECORDS

The only way to know exactly what you eat and drink is to write it down *while you are doing it*. Get yourself a flat notebook, small enough to carry in your pocket or purse, and list *everything* you eat and drink.

Also write down exactly *how much* you ate—by ounces of meat, fish and sugared vegetables. Remember that a cornerstone of the DW program is teaching yourself to see and control just how much you take in. Once you have each week's intake in your book you can see week by week what you did differently and can note how the diet changes took off ugly fat for you.

WEIGH YOURSELF IN ONCE A WEEK

You can't keep track of your progress without an accurate scale and so I recommend that you don't try false economy here. Of course the best scale is the doctor's springless type that works on balances—the type we use in DW groups. But their cost is much too high for most people, so I simply advise you to buy as well-made a scale as you can afford, in a reputable store. Keep it in your bedroom, not in the bathroom where moisture will tend to rust its springs.

You want the scale to give you a *consistent* register of your weight. To see a true measure of your pound losses, weigh yourself once a week at the same time of day, before or after the same meal, wearing the same amount of clothes.

CHECK WEEKLY TO CORRECT ERRORS

Record your weight and date it every time you "weigh in." If you lost two pounds (or more) and have eaten according to the DW program, aim to keep it up until you reach your goal. If you did not lose any pounds:

1. Go back to your list of what you ate and drank last week. You don't have a complete list? That's your big mistake and the one you must correct for the coming week. *Get a tiny notebook. Start the list. This week write down everything you eat and drink . . . within half an hour after you've had it.*

2. If you have the list, check it closely against the Basic DW Diet (Chapter 10). *What did you eat or drink that is not on the list?* What did you eat too often? What foods did you leave out? Find these errors and decide how you will correct them during the next week.

3. Check the sizes of your portions. Did you actually weigh each portion so that you took in *only* the amount in the DW diet? If you skipped meals, you may have gotten so hungry that you could not control your portions. Maybe you took seconds, cheated "just a little." . . . *You fooled yourself, but not your scale.*

At each weighing in, go back to the Basic DW diet and the Ideal Menu patterns and compare them with what you actually did to find where you went wrong and to correct it. Work to get closer each week to the precise DW diet.

Sometimes, when you do not do well on the scale and check back to the DW Basic diet, you find that you ate only what you liked and avoided other foods there that you don't like. But they may be just the proteins or vegetables that would burn fat off fastest for *you*. Try them for a few weeks to see what they might do. When I began the diet there were many foods in it I did not like. When I saw what they did for my figure, I began to love those foods.

A NEW KIND OF SHOPPING

The foods you bring into your house are the ones you will put into your mouth. Your first line of defense, therefore, is in the store. Here are good rules for dieters:

1. Never shop when you are hungry. If necessary, chew sugarless gum while shopping to help yourself resist temptation.

2. Plan what you will buy while still at home, so that you won't be won over by displays and other "goodies." Go to the store with only a list in hand.

3. Lay in large supplies of the unlimited DW vegetables,

seafoods, the other choice proteins, and the makings for DW desserts and treats. Use fresh, frozen, canned or other processed types.

4. Learn to read labels for the ingredients used to process the foods you buy and you'll not only lose pounds but save some money. If the ingredients are printed in type too small to read (which often happens) bring along a magnifying glass. Once you learn the brands you want, the shopping will go faster.

Don't buy foods that are processed with sugars, honey, corn syrup, molasses, lactose, lactate, maltose or dextrose. These have been added for taste but they are sugars and they are fattening. Enriched white bread without these additives is not only less expensive but also less fattening. Vegetables that are naturally ripened may be less expensive and their flavor is always superior to the doctored ones. Check even the artificial sweeteners for lactose. You can use tuna packed in water or in vegetable broth and cottonseed oil—but remember to drain off the broth before you eat it.

ALWAYS SET A PRETTY TABLE

The best French chefs know that if you want to please the stomach you must first please the eye. Whenever you sit down to a meal, especially on a diet program, arrange the table attractively. Use *color* in food to make it attractive. The Diet Watchers foods that add visual pleasure will help you to stay on your diet. See what the scarlet of pimiento, the fresh green or red of pepper, the rich red of a diet cherry soda can add to your resolve. Choose the green and yellow vegetables that lend attractive color contrast to your protein dishes. Use bright cloths and gay tableware to help you enjoy your diet food.

INVEST IN A BLENDER

If you add a blender to your kitchen tools you can try many new recipes that use healthful slimming ingredients instead of the old fattening ones you have been eating.

I was a gourmet cook of the old school even before I married and the first thing I bought after my wedding was an electric mixer with all the attachments—I used it to keep myself fat. But in 1961, while I was on the Diet Watchers diet, my husband asked me what I wanted for Mothers' Day.

Inwardly I was hoping for something jazzy to wear. I'd lost 40 pounds and dreamt of a flowing black peignor—but what wife can ask her husband for something like that? "Nothing," I told him, "just to be slim."

"Okay, you won't say, so you'll settle for nothing," my husband told me. And I was willing to settle for nothing—except that he was known in our family for sending me big funny cards, and I did expect that. On Mother's Day, however, he came in with a big box. "From us to you," he announced solemnly. "With all our love."

No card? I could have whacked him. I opened the box and there was—a blender. My world shattered. To help myself lose weight, I had stashed my mixer away in my clothes closet. What kind of present was this? I said, "Thank you for your present." Then I walked pointedly to *his* closet and put it up on his shelf. "What will I *do* with it? Who *needs* it?" I told him. He was crushed, but I was mad.

Two weeks later I cooled off, took it down and brought it to my kitchen counter. I decided I would try to make the delicacies I was now looking for, using the slimming foods. And that is how the recipes in this book were born.

Today the most important utensil in my kitchen is my blender. I know that a dieter needs delicacies and the blender allows you to make them. Get one with a cup large enough to hold the amount of food you will want to blend. The new blenders have convenient handles and spouts and some are unbreakable.

GET A FEW TEFLON POTS

I use a ten-inch Teflon frypan that is deep enough to cook in, as well as for Teflon-frying delicacies. It allows the cooking of many traditional treats without the fat needed to keep food from sticking to the pan. The fat used in ordinary frypans gets absorbed into your food and you gain—nothing very good, only excess poundage. Eventually, you will amortize the cost of the new pot in the savings from the cooking fat you no longer have to buy.

I also have a Teflon poacher and love it because I can poach eggs very quickly and they come out whole. No sticking.

OTHER EQUIPMENT—OPTIONAL

If you have a cloth tape measure, make a record of your waist, arm, hip, bust, neck and thigh measurements before you start on the DW diet. You will find it exciting—and a great motivater—when you measure yourself again after you have begun to lose weight and you can see exactly how many inches have vanished.

Because I work and don't like to clean my oven any more than I must, I bought an inexpensive top-of-the-stove potato baker and use it for baking acorn squash. Just wrap the squash in aluminum foil and bake right on top. No oven cleaning or fussing.

Life doesn't begin at forty but the day you become slim.

10

THE BASIC DIET WATCHERS DIET

On the Diet Watchers program, instead of counting calories we divide foods into several classes that you will soon know by heart:

1. UNLIMITED FOODS

asparagus
beet greens
broccoli
cabbage
cauliflower
celery*
chinese cabbage
cucumber
endive
escarole
green & red pepper
lettuce
bean sprouts
mushrooms
mustard greens
parsley
pickles*
pimientos
radishes
sauerkraut*
spinach
summer squash
string beans (French style)
watercress

These unlimited foods are generally the unsugared vegetables. You can eat all you want of them at or between meals, any time of day, whenever you have a feeling of hunger. Use them to help your body burn up fats and to stop yourself from eating the fattening foods. Stuff yourself with them. They have a fresh clean flavor and usually they won't make you crave more food, as the sweets do. Eat them raw or cooked, but *without* fat or sauces (except for those made with DW recipes) and without salad oil dressing.

Notice that three items on the list have an asterisk. In Diet Watchers groups we have often found that some people lose weight faster if they cut out these items. If you can lose seven pounds the first week while eating them, and two to three pounds a week thereafter, do not eliminate them. But if you are certain that you are not deviating from the Diet Watchers program in any way, and still are not losing much, cut them out and see if you lose faster.

These unlimited foods can prevent you from eating the fattening ones if you buy them in large amounts and prepare them for easy snacking. A bowlful of cauliflower broken into bite-size flowerettes and kept crisp in a bowl in your refrigerator is a snack that will help you to lose fat rather than a sneak that will put it on for you.

Also unlimited are the following drinks. You may have them at any time of day you wish, and as much as you want, except for the tomato juice which is limited to one cup each day.

bouillon
water
carbonated beverages (the non-caloric kind)
clear soups (fat free only)
seltzer or club soda
tea
coffee (black with non-sugar sweetener)
lemon and lime drinks
one cup of tomato juice (8 ounces)

Finally, you make unlimited use of the following seasonings and sauces:

horseradish
lemon
lime
salt
pepper
paprika
mustard
vinegar
all spices
all herbs (oregano, thyme, garlic, etc.)

2. LIMITED VEGETABLES

You may eat exactly one serving each day of *four ounces* from one of the following vegetables:

artichokes
bamboo shoots
beets
brussels sprouts
carrots
eggplant
green beans (mature)
okra
onions
oyster plant
parsnips
peas
pumpkin
scallions
squash (acorn, butternut, etc.)
tomato
turnips

Vary your selection each day among the green and yellow vegetables.

At Diet Watchers we work with each person to find a unique menu plan—that is, the meal at which to take each vegetable for the greatest loss, according to the individual's body chemistry. However, you will find that having them daily for dinner only, as in the ideal menu plans, will help you take off fat.

3. FRUITS

You must have three fruits every day, and one should be a high Vitamin C fruit such as orange or grapefruit. You may eat any fruit in season *except* bananas, cherries, watermelon, dried fruits, grapes.

4. MEATS, FISH AND POULTRY

General rules:

Do not eat any meat or fish that is not named in this section.

Broil, bake or roast fish, meat and poultry. *Never fry.*

Remove all visible fat before eating.

Do not eat any gravies or sauces except those made with Diet Watchers recipes.

Eat at least five fish meals weekly, more if possible.

All meat portions (unless specified differently in a DW recipe) should weigh at least six ounces after cooking. All fish fillet portions must be six ounces cooked. In general, you will find that if you allow two ounces for raw meat and for fish with bones and skin you will arrive at the correct portion of weight after cooking. However, always weigh portions cooked, just before you serve them.

We divide all meats and fish into two groups—DW first and second choices. The division is based on the amount of fat in each. Second choice proteins have a bit more fat, but not enough to substantially affect your diet. And they do offer a wider variety of foods to select from.

FIRST CHOICE MEAT AND FISH

abalone
bass
brains
chicken (breast)
cod
finnan haddie
flounder
haddock
halibut
heart (beef)
kidney
lobster
lungs
mussels
oysters
pike
scallops
shrimp
sturgeon (fresh)
trout (brook)
weakfish

SECOND CHOICE

bluefish
bonito
butterfish
chicken
eels
kidney (beef)
mackerel
pheasant
rabbit
salmon (canned)
shad
shad roe
swordfish
trout (lake)
tuna (fresh, waterpacked, or drained if it is the type packed in vegetable broth)
turkey (light meat only)
veal
white fish

EAT FROM THE FOLLOWING MEATS *THREE TIMES WEEKLY:*

beef
frankfurters
lamb
fresh salmon
turkey—*dark meat only*
liver
steak
roast beef
hamburger

5. BREAD

We have a very simple, easy-to-remember Diet Watchers rule: You *must eat* one slice (one ounce) of enriched white bread at breakfast every day, and a second slice of the same at lunch. You need this for quick energy. But *do not eat bread at any other time of day, or any other kind of bread.* You may have it toasted or not, as a "side" food or in a Diet Watchers recipe.

Never have it buttered. If you want a spread on it (at breakfast only), use a DW fruit preserve or two ounces of cottage, farmer, pot, muenster, Swiss or ricotta cheese.

For men and teenagers: A man has two slices of enriched white bread at breakfast and two at lunch. We also may add two slices for teenagers to allow for growth, depending on their progress on the program.

6. EGGS

Limit your eggs to four to seven a week. You may have eggs cooked in the shell, poached or scrambled (without fat —see Diet Watchers techniques in the recipe section).

7. MILK

You *must* drink two glasses (16 ounces) of skim milk or buttermilk every day. If you take skim milk, use the non-fat dry solids rather than the liquid kind. You may take milk any way or time you like—at or between meals, in beverages, or as a sauce. You'll find some excellent white sauces made with buttermilk among the Diet Watchers recipes.

8. THE ABSOLUTE DON'TS

Until you reach your goal and are ready to go on maintenance, do not eat or drink any of the following:

alcoholic beverages (mixed)
beer, wine, whiskey
avocado
bacon (*or any fat*)
butter
cake
candy
chocolate
coconut
cookies
crackers
cream (sweet or sour)

- doughnuts
- French dressing
- French fries
- fried foods
- gefilte fish
- gravy
- honey
- ice cream
- jam
- jelly
- jello
- ketchup
- mayonnaise
- muffins
- smoked fish
- sugar
- syrups
- nuts
- oil
- olives
- pancakes
- peanut butter
- pies
- popcorn
- potato chips
- pretzels
- puddings
- salad dressings
- soda
- ginger ale
- cola drinks
- waffles
- yogurt
- ices

Some of these, of course, are your favorite foods, the ones you *crave*. You have to give them up entirely while losing pounds. But after you get to the Diet Watchers maintenance program you will be able to have them in satisfying amounts without gaining weight. Your body will have learned to tolerate them because its chemistry will have have been altered so that it turns them into energy instead of storing them as fat, as it does now. When you have reached your goal you will reintroduce them on a gradual basis in amounts that permit your body to burn them properly.

Meantime, however, if you browse through the recipe section, you will find that there are quite a lot of treats you can substitute, and that use the proper Diet Watchers food. Want pancakes and syrup made to help you lose weight? See page 81. There are also delicious malteds, desserts, and other goodies you will come to enjoy just as much as the fattening kind.

9. THE ABSOLUTE RULE

Do not deviate from the basic Diet Watchers diet. Do not add or substitute or subtract. Every "must" food is just that —vital for your health and your good appearance. As you see, the Diet Watchers eating plan is not a "dietetic" or "restricted" one although we do cut out many foods while you are on the reducing program.

We repeat that while many physicians send patients to us, Diet Watchers does not accept new members who have a health problem without a doctor's written approval, and for your own protection, you should do no less.

Once you have his go-ahead, eat *all* the foods from this general diet in the pattern of the Ideal Menu Plans.

A girl who eats vegetables and fish turns into a cute little dish.

11

IDEAL MENU PLANS

Here is a week of eating on the Diet Watchers program. You'll see that you eat well. You won't starve, feel hungry or have to deprive yourself of treats. You can live happily while losing your ugly fat, and will use this ideal pattern as the foundation for healthful proper eating all the rest of your life, when you go on maintenance.

As it happens, the week below is an actual menu I followed when I lost my pounds. I have made one change: I used to carry a Little Care package with me for lunches, and I have substituted dishes you can get at any restaurant today (at that time they were much harder to find) or make at home.

Start with the menu below. It can help you to lose up to seven pounds the first week and, if you stay on it, an average of two pounds thereafter each week. (Naturally you will lose smaller amounts as you approach your goal). At Diet Watchers we rearrange patterns for individuals to allow for their preferences and needs, and as we observe each person's weekly fat losses, for every person has a different body chemistry. But we never cut portions or deviate from the basic general diet. You may not lose quite as much as we do in our groups, but you will reach your goal.

Carefully study the ideal week's menu to note the fixed pattern of eating every day. Except for Sunday, the time of your three main meals is the same each day of the week. You may eat your meals and snacks at a different hour than I did, but whatever your hours are, set aside a specific time of day for them and stick to this pattern doggedly. Whether you eat lunch at noon or 1 P.M. does not matter so much as setting a fixed time and following it as closely as possible, no matter where you are. You thus create a *habit* of eating at the same time each day.

The habit is valuable for several reasons. First, I find that a problem of overweight people is that their eating pattern has become so broken up that it is confused. They never know how much they eat and they rarely feel they have enjoyed a meal.

Second, a fixed pattern regulates your body chemistry in a more predictable way.

Third, a fixed pattern gives you a schedule that sets aside time for *you*. And why not? Aren't you important? A fixed pattern was one of the secrets that made my own program successful. I think it is vital to a controlled eating program and I commend it to you.

Also note at which meals you always eat or never eat certain foods, and the food combinations. When you adapt this ideal menu to suit your personal preferences be sure to keep the following specific timings: Bread always at breakfast and lunch, never at any other time of day; eggs or cheese only at breakfast, never at any other time of day; meats only at lunch or dinner; dinner vegetables *only* at dinner. Why? Foods in certain combinations work best nutritionally and the Diet Watchers combinations are devised to give you excellent nutrition. Recipes in the Cookery section are arranged to help you eat foods in the proper Diet Watchers order and combinations.

Men and boys over 15 should add two slices of bread a day—the first at breakfast and the second at lunch—and one extra fruit each day, to be taken any time.

MONDAY
First Day

8 a.m. BREAKFAST

Tomato juice, 4 ounces
French toast (recipe on page 79), 1 slice
Coffee with milk, 1 cup

12 noon LUNCH

Tin of tuna, 3¾ ounces
Salad of beet greens, cabbage, escarole, endive, mushrooms and pimiento
1 slice bread, white enriched
Coffee with milk

3 p.m. SNACK

Coffee malted (DW recipe on page 117)

5:30 p.m. DINNER

½ Broiled chicken with pineapple* (leftover from Sunday dinner)
Bamboo shoots mixed with water chestnuts, 4 ounces
Dish of mushrooms, French-style string beans, bean sprouts mixed with Coleman's English mustard sauce
Tea with lemon, saccharin

9 p.m. SNACK

Apple* malted (DW style)

11 p.m. SNACK

Blueberries* with sweet cream, to finish milk for the day (recipe on page 110)

GOODNIGHT

* Three fruits of the day.

TUESDAY
Second Day

8 a.m. BREAKFAST

½ grapefruit*
1 Poached egg on toast
Coffee with milk

12 noon LUNCH

Tomato juice, 4 ounces
Tin of salmon (4-ounce size) with large salad of lettuce, cucumber, radishes, pimiento, Chinese cabbage
1 slice bread, white enriched
Coffee with milk

3 p.m. SNACK

Strawberry* malted, DW style

5:30 p.m. DINNER

Steak (6 ounces) broiled with mushroom caps (recipe on page 96)
Brussels sprouts, carrots and peas, 4 ounces combined
Broccoli, side dish
Spinach, side dish
Fresh Pineapple,* ½ cup

9:30 p.m. SNACK

Malted (finishing milk for the day)
DW gel

11:30 p.m. BEDTIME SNACK

Mixed bowl of French-style string beans, bean sprouts, mushrooms
Diet soda, 1 glass

GOODNIGHT

* Three fruits of the day.

WEDNESDAY
Third Day

8 a.m. BREAKFAST

½ small cantaloupe*
Cottage cheese, ¼ cup
Toast, 1 slice white enriched
Coffee with milk

12 noon LUNCH

Shrimp on bed of lettuce, cucumber, green pepper, radishes, celery and pimiento
Toast, 1 slice white enriched
Coffee with milk

3 p.m. SNACK

Fresh apple*

5:30 p.m. DINNER

Marinated swordfish (recipe on page 88), 6 ounces
Tomato slices, 2 ounces
Beets, 2 ounces
Side dishes of summer squash, broccoli
Salad of escarole, shredded red cabbage
Coffee with milk
Gel with whipped cream topping (DW style)

10 p.m. BEDTIME SNACK

Ice cream (DW style) over ½ cup blueberries* (finishing milk for the day)

GOODNIGHT

* Three fruits of the day.

THURSDAY
Fourth Day

8 a.m. BREAKFAST

1 fresh orange*
1 Egg, soft-boiled
Toast, 1 slice white enriched
Coffee with milk

12 noon LUNCH

Broiled halibut, 4 ounces
Asparagus
Mushrooms
French-style string beans
Spinach
Toast, 1 slice white enriched
Coffee with milk

3 p.m. SNACK

1 pear*
Skim milk, 1 glass

5:30 p.m. DINNER

Hamburgers, six ounces
Broiled tomato (DW style recipe on page 92)
Salad of lettuce, shredded cabbage, cucumber, pimiento, celery, mustard greens, sour pickle
Diet soda
Baked apple with whipped cream

10 p.m. SNACK

Finished leftover broccoli, spinach and DW gel (nothing gets wasted)

GOODNIGHT

* Three fruits of the day

FRIDAY
Fifth Day

8 a.m. BREAKFAST

Tomato juice, 4 ounces
1 ounce grilled cheese made into DW pizza pie (recipe on page 83 includes one slice of enriched white bread)
Coffee with milk

12 noon LUNCH

Salmon, 4-ounce tin, on salad bed of lettuce, cabbage, endive, cucumber, escarole, radishes, pimiento
Toast, 1 slice white enriched
Coffee with milk

3 p.m. SNACK

Fresh apple*
Coffee malted (finishing milk for the day)

5:30 p.m. DINNER

Half of a roast chicken with stuffing (DW stuffing recipe on page 119). Whole chicken is 2½ pounds.
Bakes acorn squash, 4 ounces
Spinach
Cauliflower
French-style string beans
Mushrooms
Bean sprouts
Pimiento garnish
Relish of cranberries* and orange (DW recipe on page 104)
Gel, DW style
Diet soda

10 p.m. SNACK

Orange* sherbet

GOODNIGHT

* Three fruits of the day

SATURDAY
Sixth Day

8 a.m. BREAKFAST

Orange* juice, 4 ounces
Spanish omelet (DW style recipe on page 80)
Toast, 1 slice white enriched
Malted

12 noon LUNCH

Broiled shrimp, 4 ounces, with DW cocktail sauce (recipe on page 88) on salad of lettuce, escarole, shredded red cabbage, celery, cucumber, radishes, green pepper
Toast, 1 slice white enriched
Coffee with milk

3 p.m. SNACK

Baked apple* with DW gel

5:30 p.m. DINNER

Cream of mushroom soup, DW style (recipe on page 101)
Veal royale with carrots (recipe on pages 98–99)
Mock sweet potato pudding (recipe on page 106)
Baked butternut squash, 2-ounce portion
Stewed mushrooms
Green pepper and celery salad
Candied pineapple*
Diet soda

9 p.m. OUT FOR EVENING

Bloody Shame 1 bottle Tab

1 a.m. BEDTIME SNACK

Dish of mixed Bean Sprouts, mushrooms, Chinese cabbage, French-style string beans mixed with Coleman's English Mustard
Malted, finishing remainder of milk for the day

. . . AND HAPPILY TO BED

* Three fruits of the day

SUNDAY
Seventh Day

11 a.m BREAKFAST

½ Grapefruit*
Spinach bull's eye (recipe on page 80)
Toast, 1 slice white enriched
Coffee with milk

2 p.m. LUNCH

Tomato juice, 4 ounces
Tuna chow mein (recipe on page 88)
1 slice bread, white enriched
Diet soda
DW gel

6 p.m. DINNER

Roast beef, 6 ounces sliced
Broiled mushrooms
Mock sweet potato pudding
Candied carrots, 4 ounces
Salad of lettuce, cucumber and pimiento
Diet soda
Pineapple sherbet*

8 p.m. TV SNACK: A TWO-HOUR EATING ORGY AND NOTHING FATTENING

DW gel topped with chilled whip delight (recipe on page 114)
Malted (finished milk for the day) DW style
Baked apple* topped with DW whipped cream
Cucumber cabbage mold (recipe on page 105)
Diet soda

THANK GOD FOR A PERFECT WEEK—GOOD FOOD AND NO CHEATING

* Three fruits of the day

12

FREQUENT QUESTIONS ABOUT THE DIET WATCHERS FOODS

Here are the questions new members ask most often about the food rules on the Diet Watchers program, and the answers I give them.

Q: Why *must* I eat a slice of bread at breakfast and at lunch?

A: Your body will turn the bread into sugar, giving you energy throughout the day. At dinner you have the sugared vegetable. These energy-giving foods keep you going.

Eat only enriched sliced white bread because this does not contain additives used for "taste," such as honey or butter, which add to your fat. Look at the ingredients listing on the package of the sliced white bread you buy and do not buy brands that contain sugars or fats. You'll save money, too, because these breads are usually the inexpensive brands.

Q: Why should I eat five fish meals each week?

A: Fish is very high in protein and has no fat content at all. Protein burns fat very quickly, and so the fish protein helps you to burn off your stored fat.

Q: Why two glasses of milk each day?

A: It supplies you with the calcium and vitamins your body needs to keep healthy.

Q: Why may I not use regular skim milk?

A: Mainly because I have found in Diet Watchers that we get better weight losses when we use the powdered type which we know is 100 per cent fat-free. And it's much less expensive. Many people think they won't like the taste as well, but try making it at night, and let it refrigerate so that it is very cold in the morning.

We had a blind girl in one group who was brought by her mother, and who argued that she she could not drink the powdered kind. I told her she could have the containered milk and wrote her mother a note telling her to prepare the powdered kind my way. The daughter never knew the difference. The next week I asked her if she was drinking her milk and she said, "I love it. I love the container milk." Enough said?

Q: Why do you say that not eating enough vegetables is worse than eating cake?

A: Because if you don't eat enough vegetables, you will get hungry and you will turn to cake. The vegetables are healthy. We are a rich country, but many fat people are starving nutritionally because they do not eat enough vegetables.

Q: Why do you recommend using many spices?

A: They flavor the food and make it more interesting. Remember that your tongue has taste buds for sweet, sour, salty and bitter flavors. Because they are so active and alive they will be demanding satisfaction from you. People who like sweets have active sweet buds; people who like salty things have demanding salt buds. By using various condiments you get the flavor taste you crave, which makes dieting easier for you.

Q: What's the difference between light and dark turkey meat on the DW diet?

A: The light is like chicken. The dark contains more fat and is considered a beef meal.

Q: Why eat from that list of meats three times—no more or less—every week?
A: If you have more than three you will gain because they contain fat. At the same time, you need the red meats to get essential foods not in the other proteins.

Q. Why do you limit eggs?
A: Eggs are good for you but many doctors today hesitate to allow patients to eat a large quantity of them. Because medicine has unanswered questions about the quantity, we feel it wisest to keep your intake to a moderate level.

Q. Why may I not eat bananas?
A: Quite simply—they are fattening.

Q: No cherries?
A: Too much sugar—too fattening.

Q: But watermelon?
A: Too much sugar.

Q: Not a single grape?
A: Not a single one—too much sugar.

Q: Should I take vitamins?
A: If your doctor recommends them for medical reasons, by all means take them. But this diet is so well balanced nutritionally that you get all the vitamins you need from the foods.

Insist on eating properly. If you eat like a queen, you will look like one and be treated like one.

13

MAINTENANCE

One of the best things about the Diet Watchers diet is that while losing weight you also do two other things that will be the basis for keeping your slimness forever: You learn to eat the proper foods, in a well-balanced way, and you re-educate your "appestat"—the appetite regulator in your body.

But you must be very careful not to push your "appestat" up again. You must always have "slim eyeballs," when you give yourself portion sizes. We advise Diet Watchers on maintenance never to eat fattening foods alone, only in public (that helps them to keep self-control) and to remember always that if they eat a small portion today they can have another portion tomorrow.

I urge you, when you reach your goal, to take a new picture of yourself. See the new slim you. See how easy it becomes to take "good" pictures. But most of all, give yourself a permanent record of how well you look at your proper goal, and keep at least one in your wallet or where you can see it every day. Look at it often.

Get that new wardrobe. Get all the wonderful new clothes you could not dream of before, and enjoy yourself in them. Such enjoyment is not self-indulgent. It is your right, and what is more, the investment is a wonderful inducement to remaining slim, a promise to yourself that you will keep on the proper diet you will have learned.

Your job will be to go back to some of the fattening foods you abstained from, because you won't want to keep losing pounds but to remain just as you are. However, remember that you will have to go back to these foods slowly.

In a book meant for many different people, it isn't possible to give you rules that will work for your individual body chemistry. Not all people can eat the same foods in the same-sized portions, with the same results.

We give individual attention to a person in a group going on maintenance, introducing the fattening foods very slowly and watching for reactions in the body's weight. A person who absorbs a fattening food well turns it into immediate energy, and does not show a weight gain. A person who does not absorb fat well, shows an *immediate jump.* He cannot take the food at that time. Therefore, we set it aside and introduce other foods, again watching to see what happens.

When you create your own maintenance pattern you must work with your own body as you would with a newborn baby. You introduce foods to a baby slowly and cautiously, going from formula to skim or whole milk, to cereals and, when these are tolerated, to desserts—and from there to chicken and assorted meats. This is the careful procedure we use in trying out fattening foods on people at Diet Watchers.

We allow a full year for introducing fattening foods and careful watching to see what happens. We find that as time goes on, a diet watcher on maintenance can eat more of the fattening foods, for his body has a greater ability to deal with them. If a person stays with us on mantenance for a full year, he also learns to "see" himself as a slim person, to enjoy all the fun in living that comes to a slim person, which is a great incentive to proper eating for the rest of his life.

The important thing to remember for maintenance is this: *There is no magic outside of a proper diet.* Like me, you may have taken off and put on a thousand pounds in your lifetime career of dieting. Now you have a real chance of developing a new maintenance pattern that keeps you slim. for the rest of your life, using the Diet Watchers diet as your foundation for proper eating. *Dieting is for a short time only, but maintenance is forever.*

If you eat sweets you take up two seats.

14

DIET WATCHERS COOKERY

Here are my own favorite Diet Watchers recipes and the ones most liked by men and women in our groups. These dishes are delicious, nourishing and filling as family meals. Many also are gourmet eating that can add excitement to a party. But most important, they help you and your family to burn up ugly fat and keep you healthy. They are *easy* recipes. They are simply "different" from the ones you habitually use, the fattening ones that your mother perhaps taught you or that you read in ordinary cookbooks.

Learn them and you will add delightful, healthful dishes to your repertoire. Give your children a taste for them and you give them the priceless heritage of liking the foods and cookery that can keep them slim all their lives.

Add your own dishes that fit the Diet Watchers program. A simple delicious steak (without butter, of course), salads and other good simple recipes abound in the ordinary cookbooks. In our book you will find unique ways of enjoying many treats you crave—the kind that may have been your undoing. Now made with Diet Watchers foods and in our way, they help you lose pounds.

HOW TO USE THE RECIPES

Because this isn't an ordinary cookbook, we have not arranged the recipes according to foods in the ordinary manner but in meal-planning groups. Our arrangement makes it easy for you to plan meals as you put yourself on the Diet Watchers program. Observe the following rules:

1. Eat dishes as described *only* for the meals given. Remember that the time of day when you take in certain foods

affects your body chemistry, and on the Diet Watchers program we are altering that chemistry by food and timing so that it burns off fat most quickly. When a dish may be eaten at either lunch or dinner, we say so.

2. The ANYTIME recipes may be eaten at any meal, any time of day, or used for snacks and treats. Many are also unlimited foods. Fill yourself up with them. Enjoy them without guilt or worry.

3. Check the FESTIVE SEASON section for a delicious Diet Watchers glazed turkey with stuffing and all the "traditional" trimmings. You'll even find matzoh brie recipes—for the Passover season or whenever you feel nostalgic or ecumenical.

4. Memorize the COCKTAIL TIME section for what-to-order or prepare for yourself when the rest of the crowd is drinking. You'll enjoy the DW drinks and won't cause trouble for your host or look "different." And remember: Dieting is only temporary!

You either eat to live, or live to eat. If you live to eat, you eat with your eyes and your nose. You see it, you want it. You smell it, you eat it. (Anything close to your nose is just as close to your mouth.) And you'll be fat all your life.

BREAKFAST STARTS THE DAY RIGHT

Always begin your day with a real breakfast. This includes a fruit, one egg *or* two ounces of cheese (you can mix cheeses, if you like), one slice of bread, and a cup of coffee. You can have milk if you like. Men and boys over fifteen eat two slices of bread. Remember that you must have bread at breakfast for the immediate energy it gives you and because it helps you to control the craving for a fattening midmorning snack.

Do not use these dishes for lunches or dinner. Those meals must give you higher amounts of proteins.

Eat breakfast soon after you get up, no matter what time of day that happens to be. Some people work evenings and get up at 1 a.m. Therefore, the first meal they have after that is their breakfast.

QUICKIE EGG

1 egg
1 slice white enriched bread
Pinch salt

Toast bread. Poach egg in Teflon egg-poacher. Place egg on the slice of toast and enjoy.

FRENCH TOAST

1 egg
Pinch cinnamon
Liquid non-sugar sweetener to taste
3 tablespoons milk
1 slice enriched white bread
No-Cal cherry syrup

Mix all ingredients (except syrup) in a bowl and place bread in the mixture. Turn slice carefully so that it soaks up all liquid. Heat Teflon fry pan and on a medium flame, Teflon-fry one side. When bottom is brown, turn and Teflon-fry other side. Presto: French Toast. Top with No-Cal cherry syrup.

Or: Broil in aluminum foil under the broiler (far from flame), turning to brown both sides.

SPANISH OMELET

1 small can sliced mushrooms, drained
1 egg
½ green pepper, diced fine
Celery stalk, diced fine
Pinch oregano
Pinch salt
¼ cup tomato juice

In a deep bowl, beat all ingredients with a fork. Heat Teflon fry-pan. Pour in mixture. Brown well on one side, turn carefully and brown other side.

BULL'S EYE SPINACH RING

1 box frozen leaf spinach, drained well
1 egg
½ green pepper, diced
1 can mushrooms, drained and sliced
Pinch garlic powder
Parsley
Paprika

In a Teflon pan, place spinach in a circle and on top add diced pepper and mushrooms. Sprinkle garlic powder and salt over all. Cover pan and heat about five minutes. When hot, remove cover, crack egg in center of pan. Sprinkle a little salt and parsley on yolk of egg, and paprika on white, for color garnish. Cook uncovered until done. A filling breakfast.

BREAKFAST PUDDING

1 slice white enriched bread
1 cup skim milk
1 egg
2 tablespoons liquid non-sugar sweetener
Pinch of salt

Cube bread into a small pyrex dish. Warm the milk (do not boil). Beat egg well with hand mixer or electric beater, adding the sweetener, salt, and warmed milk as you beat. Pour mixture over the bread in the pyrex bowl and improvise a double boiler effect by placing the pyrex dish into a larger pot half filled with water. Bake in 325° F. oven for about 35 minutes. If you have a double boiler you can use that in the oven, but the pyrex dish improvisation enables you to make several at a time, cover with aluminum foil, and freeze. You can reheat on top of the oven right in the pyrex dish.

This recipe equals one glass of milk for the day.

DW CHEESE DANISH

1 slice enriched white bread
Liquid non-sugar sweetener
A little cinnamon
2 ounces cottage cheese
Powdered saccharin.

Cut crust off bread (and nibble the crust). On a piece of aluminum foil, roll out the slice of bread until quite thin, using a rolling pin or a bottle. Sprinkle a few drops of liquid sweetener and cinnamon over cheese and mix. Place cheese mixture on bread and fold in half like a clam. Pinch ends together to close tightly. Broil lightly on one side and turn to broil other side lightly brown. Sprinkle with powdered saccharin, which looks just like confectionary sugar. Enjoy every bite.

BLUEBERRY PANCAKES

1 egg
1 slice white enriched bread
¼ cup skim milk
Pinch of cinnamon
Liquid non-sugar sweetener to taste
½ cup blueberries

Blend all ingredients except blueberries in blender. Pour batter into mixing bowl and add blueberries. Heat Teflon frypan and pour in the mixed batter. Fry on one side until done. Flip over carefully and fry other side.

I suggest that you make small (four-inch) pancakes so that you can fit three into a ten-inch pan at one time, and stack them there to keep warm.

To serve, stack as traditional wheatcakes and, if you like, top with a little No-Cal diet syrup—any flavor you like (orange, raspberry, cherry, strawberry, etc.).

Subtract ¼ cup of milk for the day.

One-half cup berries equals one fruit for the day.

For variation, try STRAWBERRY PANCAKES. Make exactly as above but instead of blueberries use ½ cup sliced fresh or frozen strawberries.

APPLE PANCAKES

1 medium-sized apple
Pinch of cinnamon and liquid non-sugar sweetener mixed to taste
1 egg
¼ cup skim milk

Slice peeled apple quite thin and simmer with lemon juice, cinnamon and liquid sweetener until apple is tender. Blend the egg, bread and skim milk in blender and pour batter into mixing bowl. Add the cooked apple. Heat 10-inch Teflon pan and pour in batter to make four-inch cakes. Brown well, flip carefully to brown other side. Top with No-Cal syrup (cherry, strawberry, orange, etc., as desired).

Subtract ½ cup milk for the day.

The apple equals one fruit for the day.

SPINACH PANCAKE

Chopped spinach, drained well (1 can or 1 frozen package)
1 egg
Salt
Pepper
1 slice enriched white bread, toasted and made into crumbs

Mix all ingredients. Preheat Teflon pan and Teflon-fry, browning very well. Turn carefully to brown other side.

"POTATO" PANCAKE

1 egg
1 slice enriched white bread
Pinch salt
Pinch pepper
1 box frozen cauliflower, or fresh, overcooked until very soft
½ cup skim milk

Toast bread and put into blender to make bread crumbs. Beat egg. With fork mash cauliflower very fine so there are no lumps. Mix all ingredients and seasoning. Heat Teflon pan and with a tablespoon, spoon in each pancake. Brown on one side until golden, turn and brown other side.

If you like potato pancakes with sour cream, top with ½ cup skim milk. This is a filling breakfast for Sunday mornings.

DW PIZZA PIE

1 slice enriched white bread
1 ounce Muenster or Swiss cheese
Garlic powder
Pinch of oregano
2 teaspoons tomato juice

Broil one side of bread and turn over. Place cheese on unbroiled side and top with seasonings. Pour tomato juice over all and broil until cheese is melted.

Crazy to have pizza pie for breakfast? Try it. You'll be crazy like a slim fox!

LUNCH ONLY

Prepare these dishes *only* for lunch because they include one slice of enriched white bread, giving you sugar for quick energy, and they never include a sugared vegetable. Men and boys over fifteen need two slices of bread. These recipes also allow you 3¾ ounces of protein—the proper lunch portion on the Diet Watchers program.

Never skip lunch or you'll get so famished that you will surely go off the diet for snacks, or at dinner. Never allow more than four hours to go by between breakfast and lunch.

Many dishes here are available at restaurants. If for any reason you cannot find them, learn to carry a Diet Watchers Little Care package (see page 44). If you are cooking lunch for yourself at home, arrange the table attractively, and be sure to break into your work for a real sit-down meal.

TUNA CROQUETTES
(serves one)

1 slice bread
3¾ ounces tuna
Green pepper (diced finely)
Celery (diced)
Mushrooms (diced)

Toast bread and put in blender to make bread crumbs. Mix half of crumbs with fish, green pepper, celery and mushrooms. Make flat patty and cover top and bottom with bread crumbs. Broil on tinfoil close to flame on one side, turn carefully to broil other side until brown. Garnish with lemon wedges.

SPECIAL TUNA CASSEROLE

1 slice white enriched bread, toasted
½ broccoli bunch (fresh), or ½ box (frozen)
½ cauliflower, or ½ box (frozen)
3¾ ounces tuna fish
4-ounce can of mushrooms, drained
8 ounces skim milk
Pinch black pepper

Put toast through blender to make breadcrumbs. Combine cooked broccoli and cooked cauliflower in deep casserole dish. Add tuna. Put the mushrooms, milk and a pinch of black pepper through the blender and blend well to make a creamed mushroom sauce. Pour over vegetables and tuna in baking dish. Sprinkle bread crumbs on top and bake for 40 minutes in 350° F. oven. Absolutely delicious. Prepare it for Saturdays when you want something unusual.

SALMON CUTLETS

1 slice bread
3¾ ounces salmon
Green pepper, celery, mushrooms—all finely diced

Toast bread and put in blender to make bread crumbs. Mix half of crumbs with the salmon and diced vegetables and form into two flat patties. Cover tops and bottoms with the rest of the bread crumbs. Broil on tinfoil close to flame. Turn carefully to brown the other side. Garnish with lemon wedges.

CODFISH CAKES

3¾ ounces codfish
¼ cup water
One whole green pepper (fiinely diced)
Pinch dehydrated parsley
Pinch paprika
Pinch black pepper
Pinch garlic powder
1 stalk celery, diced
Mushrooms, diced
1 slice bread

Poach or cook codfish in water with the diced green pepper, parsley, paprika, black pepper and garlic powder. Dice the stalk of celery and mushrooms into mixture. When fish is tender (about ten minutes on medium flame) strain liquid; cool and mash fish with fork. Toast bread and blend to make bread crumbs. Mix in half of crumbs and form into patties. Sprinkle top and bottom with rest of crumbs and broil on tinfoil close to flame until brown. Turn carefully to brown other side.

LUNCH OR DINNER

You may use these dishes for either meal because the recipes do not include bread. However, note that when you have them for lunch you may use only the unlimited vegetables, and you must add a slice of white enriched bread on the side (two slices for men and boys over fifteen).

At dinnertime add a four-ounce portion of a sugared (limited) vegetable.

Also note that at lunch you eat a 3¾-ounce portion of protein and at dinner the portion is usually six ounces cooked. Where it is not possible to weigh the meat or fish by itself after cooking, the recipe tells you the raw weight, or meat-and-vegetable weight, that makes one dinner portion. Do not eat bread at dinner.

BROILED CHICKEN WITH PINEAPPLE

1 broiler, about 2½ pounds
Paprika
1 large clove garlic
¼ cup soy sauce
2 tablespoons lemon juice
⅛ teaspoon garlic powder
½ pineapple cut into chunks

Rub chicken with paprika and garlic. In broiling pan, mix the soy sauce, lemon juice and garlic powder. Place chicken in this marinade sauce for two hours, turning to immerse each side. Broil with pineapple chunks for twenty minutes on one side, then turn chicken over on other side and broil for another 20 minutes or until chicken is very brown. Keep chicken in center of broiler to avoid burning.

One-half pineapple equals one fruit.

One-half broiler equals one portion. Surprised?

SALMON LOAF

Can of salmon (7 ounces), drained
4 ounces onions, diced fine
1 can sliced mushrooms
1 green pepper, diced fine
1 stalk celery, diced small
½ cup tomato juice
Pinch parsley
Paprika
Garlic powder

Thoroughly mix the onion, mushrooms, green pepper and celery with the salmon and place in a baking dish. Shape into a square or oval form. Pour tomato juice over it, add parsley, paprika, garlic powder and bake in 350 degree oven until loaf is brown.

Six ounces equals one dinner portion and one vegetable. To use as lunch, cut out the onion and eat 3¾ ounces.

BROILED SCALLOPS

1 pound scallops
Paprika
Parsley, dehydrated
Garlic powder
⅓ cup tomato juice
Salt
Water to cover

Wash scallops thoroughly. Boil salted water and drop in scallops for five minutes. Drain well and sprinkle with paprika, parsley and garlic powder. Place on broiler rack. Preheat broiler and pour tomato juice over the scallops. Place broiler on second rack from the top. Broil five minutes or until brown, turn and brown other side.

Six ounces equals a dinner portion.

Three and ¾ ounces equals a lunch portion.

ITALIAN BAKED SCALLOPS
(A delicacy)

1 pound sea scallops
⅛ teaspoon garlic powder
Pinch paprika
1 tablespoon chopped parsley
Pinch oregano
½ cup tomato juice
½ pound fresh mushrooms
4-5 Italian frying peppers

Wash scallops. Place in baking dish and sprinkle with paprika, parsley, oregano. Pour tomato juice into a saucepan and add chopped parsley, paprika, oregano, garlic powder. Bring to a boil, lower flame and let simmer six minutes, covered. Stir when thickened. Pour over scallops. Preheat 350° F. oven. Around scallops arrange fresh mushrooms and Italian frying peppers, halved and cleaned. Bake for ½ hour or until scallops are done.

Three and ¾ ounces cooked scallops is lunch portion.

Six ounces cooked scallops equals a dinner portion.

SHRIMP SALAD

Shrimp, fresh or frozen
Lettuce
Radishes
Cucumber, scored and sliced
Pimiento strips

Boil shrimp; devein and season with DW Cocktail sauce.* Place on a large bed of lettuce with other vegetables.

Three and ¾ ounces of cooked shrimp equals a lunch portion.

Six ounces cooked shrimp equals a dinner portion.

MARINATED SWORDFISH

2 pounds swordfish
⅔ cup soy sauce
1 teaspoon grated lemon peel
2 teaspoons regular mustard
1 clove garlic, cut up very fine (or ⅛ teaspoon garlic powder)

Place fish in shallow baking pan. Mix all other ingredients in bowl and pour over fish; marinate three hours. Pre-heat broiler and broil five minutes on each side—close to flame. Garnish with lemon wedges and parsley for attractive color. This makes six dinner servings or eight lunch portions. Try it for the whole family and have some left over for lunches.

TUNA CHOW MEIN

3¾ ounces tuna, drained
½ can bean sprouts
½ can mushrooms
1 green pepper, diced
2 stalks Chinese cabbage, sliced
½ can French-style string beans (save liquid)
Coleman's dry English mustard
Soy sauce

Place tuna in strainer and wash with warm water for about two minutes. Break into chunks and combine with all the vegetables. Heat, using liquid from the French-style string

* For DW Cocktail sauce: Combine and chill ¼ cup tomato juice, 1 tablespoon white horseradish, 1 teaspoon lemon juice, ½ teaspoon chopped parsley and 1 teaspoon liquid sweetener.

beans. Drain and serve, adding Coleman's dry mustard and two drops of soy sauce.

This recipe also makes a delicious LOBSTER CHOW MEIN, SHRIMP CHOW MEIN or CHICKEN CHOW MEIN. Remember that 3¾ ounces of sea food or meat makes a lunch portion and six ounces makes a dinner portion. If you like, add four ounces of water chestnuts as a dinner vegetable only.

DINNER ONLY SOUPS AND VEGETABLES

These dishes use foods that are limited on the Diet Watchers program. Have them only at dinner. Four ounces always equals a dinner portion, and remember to weigh your portions after cooking. If you eat them raw, you get the same size portion—but more nutrients.

You may add all the unlimited vegetables you want—broccoli, cauliflower, cabbage and any others from the list in the Basic Diet to fill yourself up. You may also add soups and side dishes from the anytime recipes, but remember that *anytime does not always mean unlimited.* Whenever you eat an anytime food, keep aware that you must subtract the amounts of the limited foods in them from the allowed portion for the day.

CREAM OF SPLIT PEA SOUP WITH NOODLES

4 ounces green peas, fresh, canned or frozen
1/3 cup skim milk
1 can bean sprouts, drained
Pinch salt
Pinch pepper
Pinch dehydrated parsley
Pinch paprika
Garlic powder

Put peas into blender for five seconds (should be thick). Add milk to blender. Pour into saucepan and heat slowly. Add bean sprouts. Season with salt, pepper, the parsley, and a pinch of paprika. Add a pinch of garlic powder if desired. Heart-warming on a cold night.

This recipe equals one dinner vegetable and 1/3 cup milk.

ACORN SWEET POTATOES
(A Quickie)

1 acorn squash
Pinch cinnamon
Granulated saccharin (or liquid non-sugar sweetener)

Cut the acorn squash in half and scoop out the seeds. Sprinkle a bit of cinnamon and the non-sugar sweetener over the inside. Wrap in tin foil and bake in 400 degree oven for $\frac{3}{4}$ hour, or on top of the stove in a potato baker for $\frac{3}{4}$ hour or until soft.

Four ounces equals a dinner vegetable portion.

APPLE-BEETS

1 can beets
½ cup instant apple sauce
Pinch salt
Dash nutmeg

Mash beets with potato masher. Stir in apple sauce, salt and nutmeg. Heat until bubbly and serve. Delicious with turkey, chicken or veal. (To make instant apple sauce, put one pound of apples through blender with ½ cup cherry diet soda and a pinch cinnamon).

This recipe equals one dinner vegetable and one fruit.

CANDIED CARROTS

Carrots
Diet cherry soda
Pinch cinnamon

Pare carrots and cut diagonally into thin slices. Add enough diet cherry soda to cover carrots in saucepan and sprinkle a little cinnamon on top. Cook for 30 minutes or until carrots are soft. (Save the cooking juice for future cooking with carrots; it lasts a week refrigerated.)

Tastes just great with chicken.

Four ounces equals your dinner portion.

PICKLED BEETS AND ONIONS

4 ounces sliced beets and onions mixed
1 teaspoon pickling spices
⅓ cup vinegar
2 teaspoons liquid non-sugar sweetener

Steam the beets and onions five minutes or less. In a separate pot mix the pickling spices, vinegar and sweetener. Bring to boil, strain, and add vinegar or liquid sweetener to taste, if desired. Pour over the beets and onions and marinate overnight.

For variety, try the same recipe using only sliced onions or beets alone (using a four-ounce portion per serving).

SOUTHERN TOMATO SURPRISE

Medium-sized tomato
Cinnamon
Liquid non-sugar sweetener to taste

Cut tomato in half. On top, sprinkle cinnamon and a few drops of liquid sweetener and broil far from the flame. If you prefer cherry-flavored tomato, use some cherry No-Cal syrup instead of the liquid sweetener.

PUMPKIN CUSTARD

1 envelope plus 1 teaspoon unflavored gelatine from a second envelope
2 cups skim milk
1 pumpkin (1 pound), fresh or canned
½ teaspoon allspice
1½ teaspoon cinnamon
4 teaspoons liquid non-sugar sweetener

Dissolve gelatine in ½ cup milk. Pour rest of milk into saucepan and bring to a boil. Add gelatine and stir until dissolved. Add pumpkin, spices, sweetener. Mix well and put into bowl. Refrigerate 2 hours. Beat with electric beater until smooth.

One half cup equals four ounces of a dinner vegetable and ½ cup of milk.

SWEET POTATO PIE (PUMPKIN)

1 pound canned pumpkin
¼ cup diet black cherry soda
Pinch cinnamon
Pillsbury Orange Funny Face

Mash pumpkin fine in the cherry soda and place in a shallow baking dish. Sprinkle a little orange Funny Face and cinnamon over the top. Bake in 350° F. oven until it is bone dry and lusciously brown on top.

Four ounces equals one dinner vegetable.

ZUCCHINI WITH MUSHROOMS

1 fresh zucchini, or 1 box frozen
4 ounces tomato juice
Dash parsley, dehydrated
Dash oregano
Dash garlic powder
1 can mushrooms, drained

Bring tomato juice to a boil with all condiments in it. Add zucchini and simmer until tender. Add drained mushrooms and continue simmering five minutes.

Four ounces of zucchini equals one dinner vegetable. Mushrooms are unlimited.

ZINGY BARBECUE CATSUP

½ cup tomato juice
1 ounce diced onion
1 teaspoon liquid non-sugar sweetener
Pinch ground cloves
Pinch allspice (ground)
Pinch cinnamon
Pinch dry mustard
Garlic powder to taste
Pinch bay leaf
Pinch crushed red pepper (hot type)
3 teaspoons vinegar

Boil all ingredients in saucepan on a low flame until thickened. Chill well in refrigerator for a delicious dressing over meat, fish, vegetables and salads.

This recipe equals ½ cup tomato juice and one ounce of dinner vegetable for the day. If you omit the onion and substitute a pinch of oregano, it becomes an anytime (but not unlimited) dressing.

DINNER ONLY

These recipes are for dinner only because of their portion sizes, and because they are made with a sugared vegetable. Most are chicken, fish, turkey or veal dinners. It seems a shame to use elaborate cooking for your three weekly beef meals because you undoubtedly will prefer simple roasts, or broiled steaks or hamburgers, and these need no additions but the seasonings you like. (Frankfurters make good beef dinners, too, and don't need recipes).

Use lean beef, in six-ounce portions when cooked, and cut away any fat you can see. Add four ounces of your favorite limited vegetable plus all you want of the unlimited foods to make a gourmet meal.

The recipes below are my favorites, however, because they are delicious, and give me my slim figure. Do not fail to note ingredients that use up part of the milk, fruit, or sugared vegetable allowed for the day. Each recipe tells you how much to subtract.

Never eat bread or crackers of any kind at dinner on the Diet Watchers program. You will find it surprisingly easy to control your dinner eating if you have eaten a Diet Watchers breakfast and lunch, taken milk or fruit or a Diet Watchers snack at midday, and not allowed more than five or six hours since lunch.

CHINESE CHICKEN STEW

3½ to 4 pound chicken
1 medium onion (2 ounces) sliced
2 ounces chopped bamboo shoots and water chestnuts combined
1 cup mushrooms, drained and sliced
3 tablespoon soy sauce
1 cup bean sprouts, drained

In a shallow pan, cover chicken with water. Add onion and simmer until tender, about 2–2½ hours. Add bamboo shoots, water chestnuts, sliced mushrooms and soy sauce and continue cooking. Add small amounts of water as needed. When chicken is almost done, add the canned bean sprouts (just to heat).

BAKED FISH

½ pound haddock
Pepper
Lemon juice
Paprika
Dehydrated parsley
2 ounces onion, chopped or diced
2 ounces tomato, sliced
½ cup tomato juice
1 can mushrooms, drained
1 can bean sprouts, drained

Season haddock with pepper, lemon juice, paprika and parsley. Line bottom of a baking pan with the onion and sliced tomato. Lay fish over them. Cover with tomato juice. Circle fish with mushrooms. Bake in 350° F. oven for about 45 minutes. Ten minutes before removing fish from oven, top the mushrooms with bean sprouts.

This recipe is also delicious when made with swordfish or codfish.

STUFFED PEPPER

Green peppers
1 can sliced mushrooms
1 can (7 ounces) salmon
2 ounces onion, diced
½ cup tomato juice
Pinch parsley
1 can bean sprouts

Cut top off pepper, scoop out seeds and wash and drain. Mix salmon, diced onion and sliced mushrooms well and stuff into the pepper. Place in baking pan, adding tomato juice and parsley. Bake in 350° F. oven for ½ hour or just until pepper is tender. About ten minutes before removing, drain bean sprouts and arrange them in the tomato juice around the peppers. To serve, garnish with lemon slices.

One seven-ounce can of salmon equals a dinner portion. This recipe also equals ½ cup of tomato juice and two ounces of a dinner vegetable. (You can add two ounces of sliced tomato to equal one full dinner vegetable.)

BROILED SEAFOOD CAKES

2 cups finely chopped cooked shrimp
2 tablespoons chopped parsley
1 tablespoon chopped fresh dill or dried dill seeds
¼ cup buttermilk
Pinch salt and pepper to taste
1 tablespoon powdered dry skim milk

Mix fish with seasonings and herbs. Add buttermilk to enable you to shape the mixture into three-inch cakes. Dip cakes into powdered dry skim milk. Place cakes in broiler close to flame and broil lightly. Turn carefully to broil other side.

Six ounces cooked equals one dinner portion.

This recipe also equals ⅓ cup milk for the day.

BROILED STEAK WITH MUSHROOM CAPS

Steak, any cut you prefer
1 pound fresh mushrooms
Paprika

Break caps from mushrooms and wash thoroughly to remove sand. Sprinkle paprika on bottom of caps. Place steak on broiler and arrange mushrooms around it. Broil on one side, turn and brown other side, also turning the mushrooms when brown. Serve immediately.

I love this with tenderloin because there's no bone and so little fat to cut away, but it's good with any steak.

Six ounces steak cooked, without bone, equals your dinner portion.

BAKED STUFFED FLANK STEAK

1 flank steak cut to 8-ounce portions raw. For each 8-ounce portion, use:
½ green pepper, diced
4 ounces onion, diced
½ large can mushrooms, drained and diced
1 clove garlic, diced, or ⅛ teaspoon garlic powder
1 chicken bouillon cube
¼ cup water

Steam the pepper, onion, mushrooms, garlic and bouillon cube in ¼ cup water until tender. Spread mixture on each portion of flank steak and roll up. Skewer every two inches across finished roll. Sprinkle garlic powder on outside of roll and bake at 350° F. on a rack in an uncovered roasting pan for one hour. If you like, also sprinkle parsley and paprika on outside of roll for their appealing color.

Each stuffed steak equals one dinner portion and four ounces of your dinner vegetable.

MEAT LOAF

1 pound ground meat, lean
Pinch salt
Pinch pepper
1/8 teaspoon garlic powder
3/4 cup tomato juice

Mix all ingredients well. Mold into a square shape on a piece of aluminum foil. Place on the rack in your roasting pan, and puncture the foil to allow fat to drip down. Pour another 1/2 cup of tomato juice over meat loaf and bake in 350° F. oven one hour. Garnish with parsley.

Six ounces cooked equals one dinner portion.

This recipe also equals 3/4 cup tomato juice.

NEW SHEPHERD'S PIE

8 ounces chopped meat (beef or veal)
1/8 teaspoon garlic powder
Pinch salt
Pinch pepper
1/2 teaspoon parsley
2 ounces water
2 packages frozen cauliflower, or 1 large head, fresh
Paprika
1 chicken bouillon cube

To the meat add the garlic powder, salt, pepper, parsley and water. Mix well. Make hamburger patties and broil lightly, just long enough to drain all fat from meat. Remove and cool meat. Put through chopper or mash fine with a fork. In a saucepan, overcook the cauliflower, drain it and mash very fine with a fork. In a deep pie plate, place a layer of mashed cauliflower, covering the entire bottom and tamping it down like a pie shell. Add meat. Cover with the rest of the cauliflower and sprinkle a little paprika and parsley on top. Dissolve chicken bouillon cube in one cup water. Add four tablespoons of the liquid to the pie and bake in a 350 oven for 1/2 hour or until top crust is brown. Try this for a buffet party.

This recipe equals one eating portion.

HUNGARIAN GOULASH

½ pound stewing beef
4 ounces of combined carrots, onion, green peas
Paprika
⅛ teaspoon garlic powder
1 cup water
2 chicken bouillon cubes
½ teaspoon oregano
1 teaspoon soy sauce
1 pound fresh mushrooms
1 large green pepper, sliced into strips
1 can bean sprouts, drained

Mix all ingredients and cook one hour or until meat is done. Ten minutes before removing from flame, add drained bean sprouts. Let cool. Refrigerate. Skim off fat. Reheat and eat.

This recipe equals one dinner portion, including one dinner vegetable.

LIVER STEAK FRENCH STYLE

Beef or steer liver, ½-inch thick
4 ounces onions
1 can mushrooms, drained

Slice onions and break into rings. Place rings in Teflon pan over a small flame, cover and let simmer until soft (about five minutes). Remove cover, raise flame and brown onions. Remove them and place the liver in the hot pan, cover and on a very low flame let simmer about three minutes. Turn liver, score with a knife so that the heat penetrates; continue cooking, covered, just three minutes more. Remove cover, return onions to pan. Add mushrooms. Raise flame to highest position and quickly sear liver on both sides. It will be sweet, juicy and tender.

Six ounces of liver cooked equals a meat portion.

Four ounces of onion equals one dinner vegetable.

VEAL ROYALE

3 or 4 carrots
Thinly sliced veal, as for veal scallopini
Garlic powder
Paprika
Dehydrated parsley
1 can mushrooms (or 1 pound fresh), diced small
1 green pepper, diced
White thread or toothpick skewers
½ cup tomato juice

Peel carrots and cut in half lengthwise if thick. Season veal slices on both sides lightly with garlic powder, paprika and parsley. In the center of each veal slice place a carrot stick and top it with the diced mushrooms and green pepper. Roll veal around the vegetables, allowing carrot ends to extend on both sides. Skewer or tie with white thread. Place "birds" in the roasting pan and pour ½ cup tomato juice over them. Cover, using the roaster top or aluminum foil, and roast in a 350° F. oven for one hour.

Eight ounces of *raw* veal will be your eating portion. Weigh your carrots uncooked, too, because four ounces of carrots equals your vegetable portion.

VEAL STUFFED CABBAGE

1 head cabbage
8 ounces tomato juice
Liquid non-sugar sweetener
Lemon juice
1 pound ground veal
Pinch black pepper
½ glass water

Line bottom of a pot with cabbage leaves. Add the tomato juice, sweetener and lemon juice and bring to a boil. Taste for the sweet-and-sour flavor you prefer. To the ground veal add a pinch of black pepper and the water and mix thoroughly. Cut off core of cabbage to loosen the leaves and boil the cabbage in a separate pot until it is soft. Stuff leaves with veal. (To stuff: Place one heaping tablespoon of meat mixture at thickest end of the leaf and roll from that end until the meat is covered; with the index finger of each hand tuck in the ends toward the meat.) Place in the pot already lined with leaves and holding the flavor liquid. Cook for two hours. Refrigerate and skim off fat. Reheat to serve.

Buy inexpensive veal and ask the butcher to grind it.

Six ounces cooked in its cabbage leaf is your dinner portion.

SPARE RIBS—DW STYLE

1 large breast of veal
Paprika
Garlic
1 chicken bouillon cube
½ cup water
1 cup vinegar
¼ cup soy sauce
¼ cup lemon juice
¼ cup liquid non-sugar sweetener

Have the butcher cut through the racks of veal as in spare ribs. Rub with paprika and garlic and let stand about ½ hour. Place all other ingredients in bottom of roasting pan and mix thoroughly to dissolve bouillon cube. Marinate veal in mixture for at least three hours. Roast in 350° F. oven for 1½ hours.

Ten ounces cooked equals your eating portion.

VEAL GOULASH

8 ounces stewing veal
2 green peppers, sliced
4 ounces onion
4 ounces tomato juice
4 ounces water
Optional:
1 can mushrooms, drained
1 can bean sprouts, drained
1 clove diced garlic or pinch garlic powder
Dash paprika
Dash basil, oregano, marjoram or any spice you prefer

Cut veal into cubes or slice in strips and brown in Teflon pan. Sprinkle with paprika and any optional spices. Add the peppers, onion, tomato juice and water and simmer, covered, until soft. Refrigerate and skim off fat. Reheat to serve. The dinner portion equals six ounces of veal.

Four ounces of onion equals one dinner vegetable.

SWEET AND SOUR MEAT BALLS AND CABBAGE

1 medium-sized can tomato juice
Lemon juice
Liquid non-sugar sweetener
1 large head cabbage, shredded
2 pounds veal, ground

In a pot, combine tomato juice and lemon juice and liquid sweetener to taste. Bring to a boil and taste for a sweet-and-sour (winey) flavor as you like it. Add shredded cabbage. Dip hands in cold water to prevent sticking, and hand-roll the veal into tiny meat balls. Place them gently in the pot. Cook, covered, until meat-and-cabbage are soft (about one hour on medium flame). Cool and refrigerate. Skim off fat. Reheat to serve; it always tastes better after the second heating.

Six ounces of meat is your dinner portion. The cabbage is unlimited.

ANYTIME SOUPS

Want a bowl of hearty soup for special times when you hanker for something hot and filling? Try these, but note that only the Chinese vegetable soup (like the classic cup of hot bouillon) is also unlimited. The rest use ingredients that come from your daily allotment.

I recommend these for lunch or dinner, between meals, when you come indoors on a cold day, and while watching television. They will truly satisfy you and they are a lot more slimming than your usual coffee-and-cake routine.

CABBAGE SOUP—JEWISH STYLE

1 large can tomato juice
Lemon juice (about ½ lemon)
1 teaspoon liquid non-sugar sweetener, or to taste
½ can water (use the tomato juice can)
1 head cabbage, shredded

Bring all ingredients but the cabbage to a boil. Taste for sweet-and-sour or winey flavor you prefer. Add sweetener or lemon juice to taste. Add cabbage. Cover pot and simmer over medium flame at least 45 minutes. This can be refrigerated for two weeks.

One soupbowl equals four ounces of tomato juice.

CREAM OF MUSHROOM SOUP

½ cup skim milk
¼ cup water
½ package frozen cauliflower
1 small can mushrooms, drained
Dash dehydrated parsley
Dash papkrika

Put ½ can of mushrooms through the blender with all other ingredients except parsley and paprika and pour the resulting blended soup into saucepan. Add rest of the mushrooms and heat until boiling. Add parsley and paprika and serve.

This recipe equals ½ cup (four ounces) milk for the day.

VEGETABLE SOUP—CHINESE STYLE

1 chicken bouillon cube
1 cup boiled water
1 can bean sprouts
1 can French-style string beans
1 can mushrooms
1 leaf Chinese cabbage, cut up
½ teaspoon Coleman's English mustard

In a saucepan, dissolve the bouillon cube in boiled water, bring to a boil again, and lower flame. Add bean sprouts, string beans, Chinese cabbage and let simmer five minutes. When ready to eat, dissolve ½ teaspoon Coleman's English mustard in water and add to the soup.

Great on a cold night—and its unlimited!

TOMATO BISQUE

2 cups tomato juice
2 cups buttermilk
2 teaspoons lemon juice
1 teaspoon Worcestershire sauce
6 drops Tabasco sauce
Salt and pepper to taste

Mix ingredients and chill well. Serve in Old-Fashioned glass. Makes four servings.

Great as a soup, snack, appetizer or during the cocktail hour.

One cup equals four ounces of tomato juice and ½ cup of drinking milk.

ANYTIME SIDE DISHES AND SALADS

Add these to any meal or use them as snacks any time of day or night, when you need a pick-me-up or some help to stay on your program. Many are so good you'll want to add them to your company menus. Some are also unlimited, so what more can you ask? Some do use DW limited foods, so be sure to check the individual recipes and subtract these from your daily allotment.

INSTANT APPLE SAUCE

1 pound apples
½ cup black cherry diet soda
Pinch cinnamon

Wash and slice apples and put through blender with the cherry soda and cinnamon.

One-half cup equals one fruit.

COLE SLAW

1 cup buttermilk
1½ teaspoon lemon juice
½ teaspoon dry mustard
¼ teaspoon salt
1½ teaspoon liquid non-sugar sweetener
1 cabbage

Shred cabbage finely. Combine all other ingredients in bowl and mix thoroughly. Pour over shredded cabbage.

This recipe equals one glass drinking milk.

INSTANT CRANBERRY SAUCE

1 pound fresh cranberries, washed
½ cup black cherry soda

Put cranberries through blender with ½ cup black cherry soda and serve.

One-half cup equals one fruit.

CRANBERRY-PINEAPPLE SAUCE MOLD

1 pound instant cranberries, made as above
¼ fresh pineapple
1 envelope unflavored gelatine
No-Cal syrup—any flavor you like
1 empty can from a dinner vegetable

Cut fresh pineapple into chunks and put through blender with two or three tablespoons No-Cal syrup in the flavor you like. Heat instant cranberries, dissolving the unflavored gelatine in it. When dissolved, add the pineapple. If you happen to have an open can of a dinner vegetable, wash it, pour in mixture and refrigerate to mold. To remove from can: Put can on a plate upside down. Remove lid with a can opener and mold will slide onto the plate.

Two slices, ½-inch thick each, equals one fruit.

CRANBERRY-ORANGE RELISH

1 cup fresh cranberries, washed
½ unpeeled orange (remove seeds)
1 tablespoon liquid non-sugar sweetener

Put cranberries and the half unpeeled orange through food chopper, using perforated coarse blade. Stir in liquid sweetener and chill in refrigerator to blend flavors (½ hour). Also make by putting sweetener and orange through blender, then adding fresh cranberries and continuing to blend together until berries are pulverized. Refrigerate to blend flavors.

Perfect with chicken, turkey, veal.

One-half cup equals one fruit.

SONO'S SESAME CUCUMBERS
(An Oriental Treat)

1 large cucumber, peeled
6 to 8 red radishes (optional)
2 tablespoons white sesame seeds
1 tablespoon white vinegar
2 tablespoons soy sauce
1 drop liquid non-sugar sweetener
Pinch of salt, if needed

Slice cucumber and radishes thin. Let stand 1–2 hours. Rinse under cold water and squeeze out moisture between palms. In heavy skillet over low heat, toast sesame seeds until golden. Crush seeds in mortar bowl or with rolling pin. Mix with remaining ingredients, adding salt if needed only after tasting, as soy sauce is sometimes quite salty.

Considered as either salad or relish, you'll find these sesame-dressed cucumbers excellent with chicken, fish or shellfish. And unlimited!

CUCUMBER CABBAGE MOLD

2 envelopes unflavored gelatine
2 envelopes lemon Pillsbury Funny Face
2 cups boiling water
1¾ cups cold water
2 tablespoons vinegar
1 tablespoon white horseradish
½ teaspoon salt
1 large cucumber
1 cup cabbage, shredded

Dissolve gelatine in boiling water. Add lemon Funny Face, cold water, vinegar, horseradish and salt. Chill until partially set. Pour ½ cup of gelatine mixture into five-cup ring mold. Cut 10–15 paper-thin slices of cucumber and arrange them in the ring mold over the gelatine. Pour a thin layer of gelatine over them and chill to set. Add the cabbage and, again, a thin layer of gelatine. Chill until almost set. Dice remaining cucumber to make one cup and add it, covering with any remaining gelatine. Chill until firm. You will have alternating layers of gel, cucumber, gel, cabbage, gel, diced cucumber and perhaps gel on bottom—delicious and very pretty. And unlimited!

PICKLED FRENCH-STYLE STRING BEANS

1 can French-style string beans (or 1 box frozen)
1 teaspoon pickling spices
⅓ cup vinegar
2 teaspoons liquid non-sugar sweetener

Steam the beans five minutes or less (if frozen, follow directions on box) and strain. In a separate pot mix the pickling spices into the vinegar and liquid sweetener. Bring to a boil. Strain, taste and add vinegar or sweetener if desired. Pour over beans and let stand overnight. Unlimited.

To make PICKLED CAULIFLOWER, BROCCOLI, GREEN PEPPERS or MUSHROOMS: Simply substitute any of these for the beans and serve yourself all you want.

FRUIT SALAD SUPREME

Orange
Apple
Pear
Grapefruit
Small melon
Blueberries
Pinch cinnamon
½ cup No-Cal cherry syrup

Make small melon balls. Put into a pretty bowl and slice in all the other fruits, except blueberries. Add the No-Cal syrup, top with some blueberries and a pinch of cinnamon. Toss lightly and refrigerate.

One-half cup equals one fruit.

DIET WATCHERS RELISH

1 cup finely chopped apples
1 cup finely shredded cabbage
½ cup finely chopped green pepper
1 tablespoon chopped pimiento or red pepper in vinegar
3 tablespoons vinegar
2 teaspoons liquid non-sugar sweetener
½ teaspoon salt
¼ teaspoon ginger
¼ teaspoon dry mustard
Dash cayenne

Combine apples and vegetables. In a second bowl, combine spices, mixing well. Pour over apples and vegetables, tossing lightly. Refrigerate at least one hour before serving.

This equals one fruit. But you can have it anythime as a delicious snack.

MOCK SWEET POTATO PUDDING

3 packages (or fresh) summer squash
Diet pineapple or orange soda
Pillsbury orange Funny Face, one envelope
Pinch cinnamon

Cook the squash in a small amount of the pineapple or orange soda until soft, then put everything through the blender. Transfer to bowl, add a package of Funny Face, and mix. Pour into shallow baking pan and sprinkle some cinnamon over the top just for the wonderful aroma. Bake in 350° F. oven until bone dry.

Too delicious to be unlimited, but it is!

Stock up on Funny Face (a granulated orange flavoring) in the summer season if your stores don't carry it during the winter.

TOMATO ASPIC

8 ounces tomato juice
1 envelope unflavored gelatine
½ tablespoon mixed pickling spices
Pinch pepper
1 tablespoon lemon juice

Soften gelatine in tomato juice. Stir in the pickling spices, salt and pepper. Heat to boiling point. Simmer five minutes to blend flavors. Stir in lemon juice. Strain ingredients and pour into mold. Chill in refrigerator until firm. Unmold on crisp lettuce.

Entire recipe equals one tomato juice portion for the day.

ANYTIME DRESSINGS

Traditional rich dressings traditionally ruin figures. The following use Diet Watchers foods that help to burn fat off and they add zip to fish, salads, vegetables and leftover meats. However, they are all made with limited foods, so don't forget to account for them, in the amounts indicated in each recipe, when you total your eating for any day.

People who like sour cream may learn to like buttermilk almost as well, and they will like much better what it does for their figures. But more commonly, I find, new Diet Watchers protest, *"Buttermilk—yek! And as a dressing?"* But it's wonderful for thickening and I dress it up with condiments and spices to give it any flavor I like. It makes an excellent Hollandaise sauce and—with liquid sweetener—a terrific dressing for fruit salad.

If you are one of those who find it hard to drink two glasses of milk a day, buttermilk dressing is a great help in getting your daily milk portion.

SPICY BUTTERMILK SALAD DRESSING

1 cup buttermilk
1/4 teaspoon salt
1/8 teaspoon pepper
1/4 teaspoon dry mustard in 1 tablespoon water
1 teaspoon Worcestershire sauce
Dash of cayenne
1 tablespoon vinegar
1/2 clove garlic

Combine all ingredients in a jar. Shake vigorously and refrigerate. Before serving, remove garlic and shake vigorously again.

Delicious on leftover cold fish and salads.

One cup equals one glass of milk.

QUICK BUTTERMILK DRESSING
("Hollandaise" Sauce)

1 cup buttermilk
1/2 teaspoon lemon juice
1/4 teaspoon salt
1 1/2 teaspoon liquid non-sugar sweetener
1/2 teaspoon Coleman's mustard (dry powder)

Mix well and refrigerate.

This recipe equals one cup of drinking milk.

Try this over freshly cooked or leftover fish, hot asparagus and broccoli, or salad.

DW FRENCH DRESSING

½ cup tomato juice
½ cup vinegar
½ teaspoon dry mustard
⅛ teaspoon garlic powder
6 drops liquid non-sugar sweetener
Pinch oregano
Pinch salt and pepper to taste

Combine all ingredients and shake well in a jar with tight-fitting lid. Keep refrigerated and shake before using.

This recipe equals ½ cup tomato juice.

SEAFOOD COCKTAIL SAUCE

¼ cup tomato juice
1 tablespoon white horse-radish
1 teaspoon lemon juice
½ teaspoon chopped parsley
1 teaspoon liquid non-sugar sweetener

Combine all ingredients and chill. Delicious over cold left-over fish and salads.

This recipe equals ¼ cup tomato juice.

ANYTIME DESSERTS

These are pleasure foods. They taste either just like, or better than, the ugly fat-making, unhealthy kind you have been eating up to now. You can enjoy them at mealtimes or as in-between snacks, and you'll serve at least some of them to company, too—for a party dinner or casual "Coffee-and" entertaining. Long after you have gone on maintenance, you will keep them in your repertoire just because they are delicious treats.

Many use limited foods, so don't forget to record them. Some are unlimited—so have all the eating pleasure you want.

DIET WATCHERS BAKED APPLE

10 Rome apples

8 ounces black cherry diet soda

Core apples and peel a small crown of skin off the top. Sprinkle with a little cinnamon. Turn apples upside down and pour soda into deep fry pan. Cover pan and cook on top of stove until done.

One apple is one fruit, and it's so delicious you'll never want it any other way.

BAKED APPLE WITH SWEET CREAM

For a fabulous topping, add ½ cup buttermilk, mixed with liquid non-sugar sweetener to taste, and juice from the pan.

BLUEBERRIES AND SWEET CREAM

½ cup blueberries
½ cup buttermilk

Liquid non-sugar sweetener to taste

Wash blueberries and put into bowl. Pour buttermilk over fruit and stir in liquid sweetener to taste.

One-half cup blueberries equals 1 fruit for the day and ½ cup buttermilk equals ½ cup drinking milk.

For delicious STRAWBERRIES AND SWEET CREAM: Use the

same quick recipe but substitute ½ cup whole strawberries. And if you prefer either fruit with a "sour cream flavor," simply omit the liquid sweetener.

CANTALOUPE WITH LEMON FILLING

2 cups skim milk
1 envelope gelatine, unflavored
¼ cup liquid non-sugar sweetener
1½ teaspoons lemon juice
1 cup No-Cal syrup (any flavor)
1 cantaloupe

Pour milk into a small saucepan and sprinkle gelatine over it. Let stand three to five minutes. Stir in liquid sweetener. Heat slowly, stirring until gelatine is dissolved. Remove from heat. Stir in the lemon juice and syrup. Cut canteloupe in half and remove seeds. Chill mixture until it is thick enough to mold. Dry the center of the canteloupe with paper towelling and fill it with the thickened gelatine mixture. Chill in refrigerater until firm. When ready to eat, pour more No-Cal syrup on top of the filling.

One-half cantaloupe equals one fruit and one cup of drinking milk.

CHIFFON MOUSSE

1 envelope unflavored gelatine
⅓ cup water
⅓ cup skim milk
1 teaspoon instant coffee and non-sugar sweetener to taste, or 1 teaspoon No-Cal syrup, any flavor
3 or 4 ice cubes

Stir gelatine into water and heat until dissolved. Let cool. Put all other ingredients through the blender and add cooled gelatine. Whip until ice cubes are dissolved. Makes a full soup bowl. Refrigerate to mold.

This recipe equals ⅓ cup drinking milk.

COFFEE JELLY

1 envelope gelatine
1 tablespoon instant coffee
½ teaspoon liquid non-sugar sweetener or to taste
½ cup cold water
1 tablespoon lemon juice
1 cup boiling water

In medium bowl mix gelatine, sweetener, coffee. Stir in cold water and let stand for five minutes to soften gelatine. Add lemon juice and boiling water and stir until completely dissolved. Cool slightly and refrigerate until it is like a soft pudding. With an electric or hand beater, beat until light and fluffy, then refrigerate until firm. Unlimited.

BROILED OR BAKED GRAPEFRUIT

Grapefruit
Cinnamon
Liquid sweetener

Wash grapefruit skin and cut in half as for ½ grapefruit serving. Segment as usual. Sprinkle with cinnamon and the sweetener to taste. Broil or bake until lightly browned (15 or 20 minutes) far from flame.

This is like a carmelized treat. Delicious as appetizer, dessert or for "Coffee-and" entertaining.

One-half grapefruit equals one fruit.

CANDIED PINEAPPLE

Pineapple
Diet black cherry soda

Cut pineapple in half lengthwise, leaving top leaves on each half. With grapefruit knife, scoop out pineapple meat and cube into one-inch chunks. In a pan, cook chunks in ½ bottle of Diet black cherry soda until fruit is slightly tender (fork pierces easily). Refrigerate to chill. To serve, return pineapple chunks to shell and pour a little of the chilled cooking juice over the top.

This is beautifully decorative as an appetizer, dessert or for "Coffee-and" entertaining.

One half of a pineapple equals one fruit.

ORANGE SHERBET

3 tablespoons concentrated frozen orange juice (unsweetened)
4 ounces skim milk
5 drops liquid non-sugar sweetener

Blend together in blender and pour into four sherbet cups. Freeze one hour only.

One sherbet equals one fruit and ⅛ cup milk.

ICE POP

1 package summer squash
½ cup water
½ package Pillsbury Funny Face (any flavor you like)
Pinch of cinnamon

Boil squash in water until soft. Put the squash, water, Funny Face and cinnamon through blender. Pour into popsicle mold or Dixie cups and freeze.

Treat yourself anytime—all you want.

RASPBERRY SOFT-FREEZE ICE CREAM

½ cup cold water
½ cup raspberry No-Cal syrup
1 envelope unflavored gelatine
2 cups skim milk

Mix all ingredients and place in saucepan. Stir to dissolve gelatine, then heat until just below boiling. Pour skim milk in separate bowl; add hot mixture and stir. Pour into individual dishes, chill until stiff and eat.

One cup equals one cup of milk for the day.

RASPBERRY SHERBET

Make mixture as for soft-freeze ice cream. Then pour one cup of mixture into ice cube tray and place in freezer. When crystals form (in about five minutes) put through the blender for your raspberry sherbet.

One cup equals one cup of milk for the day.

STRAWBERRY ICE CREAM FLOAT

1 envelope unflavored gelatine
¼ cup cold water
2 cups strawberries
1 teaspoon liquid non-sugar sweetener
1 tablespoon lemon juice
⅛ teaspoon salt
1 drop red food coloring
⅓ cup dry powdered milk
¼ cup ice water

Soften gelatine in cold water and dissolve by boiling. Stir until completely dissolved. Mash strawberries. Add sweetener, lemon juice, salt, coloring and strawberries to softened gelatine. Chill until mixture begins to thicken. Combine dry milk and ice water and beat at high speed of electric or hand mixer until stiff. Fold into gelatine and spoon into cups.

One cup squals one fruit and ¼ cup of milk.

DW TOASTED ALMONDS

2 pounds fresh mushrooms

Decap the mushrooms and wash both the caps and stems. Place them on a large cookie sheet. Preheat oven 350° F. On the second rack, bake mushrooms until bone dry and crisp. Lower oven heat to 300–325° F. if mushrooms burn. Delicious exactly as is—a real treat. Keep a jarful in the refrigerator, for your witching hour, to take with you to the movies, or to serve special guests as an hors d'oeuvre.

CHILLED WHIP DELIGHT

1 envelope gelatine, unflavored
¼ cup water
½ cup lemon No-Cal syrup
2 cups buttermilk (use the thick kind)
Liquid non-sugar sweetener
1 lemon peel, grated

Mix gelatine in water. Heat syrup in pan. Mix the dissolved gelatine and syrup, then shut off the flame. Add buttermilk and sweeten to taste. Pour into mixing bowl and chill until set—about one hour. Beat well with egg-beater or electric mixer. Pour into four sherbet glasses or bowls and top with grated lemon peel, then chill in refrigerator until set again. This tastes exactly like the ice-cream parlor dessert.

This recipe may also be made with other No-Cal syrups, but without the lemon peel. We like the black cherry and raspberry best.

Each serving equals ½ cup milk.

ANYTIME TOPPINGS

Use these as toppings anytime of day or night, over desserts or other Diet Watchers dishes. Many are delicious as spreads for your breakfast or lunchtime bread, or even alone as snacks—they are that good. Just remember that they do use milk or fruits, both of which are limited—so enjoy them but account for them in your total daily eating record.

BLUEBERRY JAM

2 cups blueberries
1 cup water
1 envelope gelatine, unflavored
1 teaspoon liquid non-sugar sweetener

Dissolve gelatine in water. Add blueberries and sweetener and simmer for about 15 minutes. Place in jar and refrigerate.

One-half cup equals one fruit.

PEACH JAM
(A Summer Delight)

10 peaches
2 teaspoons liquid non-sugar sweetener
1 package gelatine, unflavored
Lemon juice if desired

Plunge peaches into boiling water for about one minute and then peel. Slice peaches and boil with liquid sweetener, the gelatine and ¼ cup water. Let cool. Taste and add lemon juice and sweetener if desired. Refrigerate overnight in a small jar. It can keep two weeks—if it lasts that long!

One-half cup equals one fruit.

DW DREAM WHIP

⅓ cup dry powdered milk
½ cup No-Cal syrup (any flavor)
⅓ cup cold water

Mix the powdered milk and syrup with cold water and beat in electric or hand beater until very fluffy. Terrific over DW gel or as a separate dessert.

This recipe equals one cup of drinking milk.

BUTTERMILK TOPPING

½ cup buttermilk

Liquid non-sugar sweetener

Sweeten the buttermilk to your taste and pour over any fruit. But remember that this equals ½ cup drinking milk.

LEMON WHIPPED CREAM TOPPING

¼ cup cold water
1 tablespoon lemon juice
⅓ cup powdered skim milk
Liquid non-sugar sweetener to taste—or about 2 tablespoons

Mix all ingredients and chill in refrigerator (including bowl and mixing beaters). Allow to chill 2–3 hours. Then beat mixture until it stands in peaks. Eat at once, just like ordinary whipped cream or use to top baked apple, gel, baked pineapple.

This recipe equals one glass milk for day.

WHIPPED CREAM TOPPING

3 tablespoons water
½ teaspoon gelatine, unflavored
1 tablespoon liquid non-sugar sweetener
⅓ cup powdered dry milk

Mix ingredients and chill in refrigerator (including bowl and mixing beaters) for 2 to 3 hours. Then beat until mixture stands in peaks.

Use as a topping for pies, custard, DW gel or fruit.

To vary the flavor, add ½ teaspoon instant coffee, or ½ teaspoon cinnamon, or ½ teaspoon lemon juice.

This recipe equals 1 glass milk.

MALTED TREATS

These delicious malteds won't add to your guilts, thicken those layers of soft fat or shorten your life. They help you to get your daily milk allotment and tone your skin and your muscles. Enjoy every drop.

FRUIT MALTED

½ cup diet soda (any flavor)
1 cup skim milk
6 thin ice cubes

Put all the ingredients through the blender and drink up.
This recipe equals one cup of drinking milk.

APPLE MALTED

1 apple
1 cup skim milk
6 thin ice cubes
Liquid non-sugar sweetener to taste

Slice apple and put through blender with skim milk, ice cubes and liquid sweetener to taste. Delicious and healthy!
This recipe equals one cup of milk and one fruit for the day.
For STRAWBERRY MALTED: Use the same recipe but substitute ½ cup of strawberries for the apple.

DIET WATCHERS COFFEE MALTED

½ cup skimmed milk
½ teaspoon instant coffee
2 saccharin tablets
6 thin ice cubes

Put milk, coffee, saccharin and two ice cubes through the blender. Add two more cubes at a time until all ice cubes are dissolved. Let blender run until malted is thick and frothy.
This recipe equals ½ cup drinking milk.

FESTIVE SEASON

What's a holiday? Certainly it's not the time to *cheat* yourself out of a good figure—and these delicious recipes for the traditional festive foods show you that there is no reason why you can't serve and enjoy them when they are prepared in a new slimming, Diet Watchers way. Included here are recipes for Christmas, Thanksgiving and Passover meals. They are so good—and good for you—you'll use them at other times too. Have a holiday all year long.

GLAZED TURKEY

1 turkey
Paprika
Garlic
Parsley, dehydrated or fresh
1 envelope Pillsbury orange Funny Face
2 glasses water

Sprinkle garlic, paprika and parsley inside and all over turkey and let stand about three hours to absorb flavors. Place turkey in roasting pan with breast up. Sprinkle orange Funny Face over entire turkey and rub into skin. Add water to roasting pan. Preheat oven and roast bird at 350° F., basting every half hour. Turn turkey completely over and continue roasting and basting until drumstick moves easily.

(Note: Many people love garlic powder for inside seasoning but you may prefer to omit it. To protect your hands from orange coloring, use clear plastic rubber gloves while rubbing bird with orange Funny Face.)

Six ounces of turkey white meat cooked and sliced equals one dinner portion. Six ounces of turkey dark meat cooked equals one beef meal.

Try this recipe also for GLAZED CHICKEN.

TURKEY STUFFING SURPRISE
(For 10-pound bird)

1 package frozen cauliflower (or 1 medium-sized head), cooked and mashed
1 can French-style string beans, drained and chopped
1 can mushrooms, drained and diced
1 chicken bouillon cube dissolved in ½ cup hot water
1 tablespoon soy sauce

Mix all ingredients well and stuff turkey. Increase amount in proportion for a larger bird. Truss and skewer, or sew bird in traditional fashion.

Delicious and unlimited!

BAKED PUMPKIN PIE

2 cups canned or fresh pumpkin, strained
1 cup skim milk
Pinch salt
2 tablespoons liquid non-sugar sweetener
½ teaspoon cinnamon
½ teaspoon ginger
¼ teaspoon nutmeg
¼ teaspoon cloves (optional)

Mix all ingredients and bake in 325° F. oven until brown.

Four ounces of pumpkin serving equals one dinner vegetable and ¼ cup milk.

STUFFED ORANGE DELIGHT

Four navel oranges
3 tablespoons concentrated frozen orange juice (unsweetened)
4 ounces skim milk
5 drops liquid non-sugar sweetener

Wash and dry oranges. Cut off a thin top slice. Scoop out orange centers in one piece, being careful not to break the outer skin. Put the concentrated orange juice, milk and liquid sweetener through the blender and pour the resulting mixture into orange shell. Freeze one hour only. When serving stuffed oranges at dessert time, set the top "cap" slice into the sherbet at a jaunty angle.

The orange center makes a spectacular garnish for main dish turkey, chicken or veal. Slice it thinly and arrange slices around the roast on the serving platter.

One stuffed orange equals one fruit and ⅛ cup milk. If you eat any of the garnish orange slices, subtract them from your fruit allotment.

PASSOVER MATZO PANCAKES
For Breakfast Only

1 egg
½ sheet matzo
¼ cup skim milk
½ teaspoon liquid non-sugar liquid sweetener

Put all ingredients through blender until fine. Heat Teflon pan or Teflon griddle. Pour batter to make small round pancakes and brown on one side; turn carefully to brown second side. To serve, top with orange No-Cal syrup. Orange and matzo make a truly yummy combination.

PASSOVER BREAKFAST: FRIED MATZO BREI
For Breakfast only

1 egg
½ sheet of matzo
¼ cup skim milk
½ teaspoon liquid non-sugar sweetener, or salt and pepper

Soak matzo for five minutes in cold water and blot dry. Beat egg, milk and sweetener (or seasoning) together. Soak matzo in the batter. Heat Teflon pan; fry on one side, flip and fry on other side. Or broil on tinfoil, turning to brown both sides. You can leave out sweetener and top with No-Cal cherry or raspberry syrup.

PASSOVER PATTIE
(Lunch Treat from the Sea)

½ sheet of matzo, put through blender
3¾ ounces of fish*
A dash of salt and pepper
Chopped green pepper and mushrooms
1 ounce tomato juice
Dash garlic powder
Dash parsley

Mix all ingredients and form into a pattie. Pour tomato juice over it and sprinkle with garlic powder and parsley. Broil on one side five minutes, then turn and broil other side five minutes.

*This recipe is delicious with flounder, codfish, halibut, whitefish, carp or any cooked leftover fish.

COCKTAIL TIME

"They" are drinking? You can, too. Nobody else really cares that much what you are having, if you follow the old rule: "Don't complain; don't explain." These are all easy drinks that you or your host can prepare using ingredients that are part of any household or bar pantry. Self-control at cocktail time is a cornerstone of your dieting. Instead of reaching for that drink, reach for your goal.

DW BLOODY SHAME ON THE ROCKS: Tomato juice on ice cubes. Add a twist of lemon. Eight ounces equals your tomato juice portion for the day.

TALL STORY WHISKEY AND SODA: Club soda on ice cubes with a twist of lemon. Liquid non-sugar sweetener makes it taste like soda.

LEMONADE: Ice water with lemon and liquid non-sugar sweetener.

LIMEADE: Ice cubes, lime juice, liquid non-sugar sweetener and a thin slice of lime.

ICED TEA OR ICED COFFEE: The way you usually make it but using liquid non-sugar sweetener instead.

DW INSTANT ICED TEA: Make tea ahead of time and freeze it in cubes in the ice cube freezer tray.

DW CHAMPAGNE: Have Diet soda in a champagne glass, any flavor you like. Cherry Diet soda is your pink champagne or wine. You'll have reason to celebrate with the real thing—after you've reached your goal and gone on maintenance.

INDEX TO RECIPES

Acorn sweet potatoes, 90
Almonds, toasted, 114
Apple, baked, 110
Apple-beets, 91
Apple malted, 117
Apple pancakes, 82
Apple sauce, instant, 103

Baked apple, 110
  with sweet cream, 110
Baked fish, 95
Barbecue catsup, 93
Beets, pickled, and onions, 91
Blueberries and sweet cream, 110
Blueberry jam, 115
Blueberry pancakes, 81
Breakfast pudding, 80
Bull's eye spinach ring, 80
Buttermilk dressing, 108
Buttermilk topping, 116

Cabbage soup, Jewish style, 101
Cantaloupe with lemon filling, 111
Carrots, candied, 91
Cheese Danish, 81
Chicken stew, Chinese, 94
Chicken with pineapple, broiled, 86
Chilled whip delight, 114
Chiffon mousse, 111
Cocktail sauce, 109
Cocktails, 121
Codfish cakes, 85
Coffee jelly, 111
Coffee malted, 117
Cole slaw, 103
Cranberry-orange relish, 104
Cranberry-pineapple sauce mold, 104
Cranberry sauce, instant, 103
Cream of mushroom soup, 101
Cream of split pea soup, 90
Cucumber cabbage mold, 105

Desserts:
  Baked apple, 110
  Blueberries with sweet cream, 110
  Candied pineapple, 112
  Cantaloupe with lemon filling, 111
  Chiffon mousse, 111
  Chilled whip delight, 114
  Coffee jelly, 111
  Grapefruit, broiled or baked, 112
  Ice pop, 113
  Orange sherbet, 112
  Pumpkin pie, 119
  Raspberry sherbet, 113
  Raspberry soft-freeze ice cream, 113
  Strawberry ice cream float, 113
  Toasted almonds, 114
Diet Watchers relish, 106
Dream whip, 115

Eggs:
Spanish omelet, 80
Quickie egg, 79

Fish:
Baked fish, 95
Codfish cakes, 85
Salmon cutlets, 85
Salmon loaf, 86
Swordfish, marinated, 88
Tuna casserole, 84
Tuna chow mein, 88
Tuna croquettes, 84
Flank steak, stuffed, 96
French dressing, 109
French toast, 79
Fruit malted, 117
Fruit salad supreme, 106

Goulash:
Hungarian, 98
Veal, 100
Grapefruit, broiled or baked, 112

"Hollandaise" sauce, 108
Hungarian goulash, 98

Ice pop, 113

Lemon whipped cream topping, 116
Liver steak, French style, 98

Malteds:
Apple, 117
Coffee, 117
Fruit, 117
Matzo brei, fried, 120
Matzo pancakes, 120
Meat loaf, 97
Meat:
Baked stuffed flank steak, 96
Broiled steak with mushroom caps, 96
Hungarian goulash, 98
Liver steak, French style, 98
Meat loaf, 97
Spare ribs, 99
Sweet and sour meat balls and cabbage, 100
Veal goulash, 100
Veal royale, 98
Veal stuffed cabbage, 99

Omelet, Spanish, 80
Orange delight, 119
Orange sherbert, 112

Pancakes:
Apple, 82
Blueberry, 81
"Potato," 82
Spinach, 82
Passover pattie, 120
Peach jam, 115
Pineapple, candied, 112
Pizza pie, 83
"Potato" pancake, 82
Poultry:
Broiled chicken, with pineapple, 86
Chinese chicken stew, 94
Glazed turkey, 118
Pumpkin custard, 92
Pumpkin pie, 119

Quickie egg, 79

Raspberry sherbet, 113
Raspberry soft-freeze ice cream, 113
Relish:
Cranberry-orange, 104
Diet Watchers, 106

Salad dressing:
French, 109
Quick buttermilk ("Hollandaise"), 108
Spicy buttermilk, 108
Salads:
Fruit, 106
Shrimp, 88
Salmon cutlets, 85
Salmon loaf, 86
Scallops, broiled, 87
Italian style, 87
Seafood:
Seafood cakes, 96

Scallops, broiled, 87
Scallops, Italian, 87
Shrimp salad, 88
Seafood cakes, 96
Seafood cocktail sauce, 109
Shepherd's pie, 97
Shrimp salad, 88
Sono's sesame cucumbers, 104
Soups:
Cabbage, Jewish style, 101
Cream of mushroom, 101
Cream of split pea with noodles, 90
Tomato bisque, 102
Vegetable, Chinese style, 102
Southern tomato surprise, 92
Spanish omelet, 80
Spare ribs, 99
Spicy buttermilk salad dressing, 108
Spinach pancake, 82
Spinach ring, 80
Steak with mushroom caps, broiled, 96
Strawberry ice cream float, 113
String beans, pickled, 105
Stuffed orange delight, 119
Stuffed pepper, 95
Sweet and sour meat balls and cabbage, 100
Sweet potato pie (pumpkin), 92
Sweet potato pudding (mock), 106
Swordfish, marinated, 88

Tomato aspic, 107
Tomato bisque, 102
Tomato surprise, 92
Toppings:
Blueberry jam, 115
Buttermilk, 116
Dream whip, 115
Lemon whipped cream, 116
Peach jam, 115
Whipped cream, 116
Tuna casserole, 84
Tuna chow mein, 88
Tuna croquettes, 84
Turkey, glazed, 118
Turkey stuffing surprise, 118

Veal goulash, 100
Veal royale, 98
Veal stuffed cabbage, 99
Vegetables:
Acorn sweet potatoes, 90
Apple-beets, 91
Beets and onions, pickled, 91
Candied carrots, 91
Cucumber cabbage mold, 105
French-style string beans, pickled, 105
Mock sweet potato pudding, 106
Pumpkin custard, 92
Sesame cucumbers, 104
Spinach ring, 80
Tomato surprise, 92
Zucchini with mushrooms, 92
Vegetable soup, Chinese style, 102

Whipped cream topping, 116

Zingy barbecue catsup, 93
Zucchini with mushrooms, 92

ACKNOWLEDGEMENTS

With deep gratitude to my husband Al Gold, my daughters Michelle and Sharyn, and to Robert D. Weissman for all their help in allowing me to create and work with Diet Watchers. Also, my thanks to my lecturers for their dedication to the people who come to Diet Watchers. In particular, I want to name Joan Albonese, Delores Austin, Edna Hradecky, Rita Presnick, Roslyn Schumer, Doris Winter and Madeline Volpe.

—Ann Gold

And my thanks to Bert Briller, to Joan and Robbie, and to Louise Siler, who so graciously allowed me to try all the new Diet Watchers recipes out on them.

—Sara Welles Briller